Contents

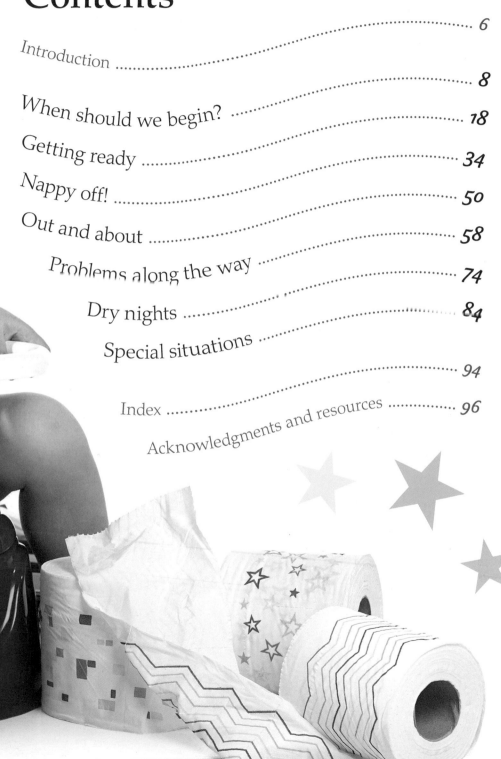

Introduction

After some two thousand nappy changes at the very least, the thought of ditching the bother, waste, and expense of nappies is likely to be hugely appealing. However, starting to potty train can feel like a big step into the unknown – what do you do, and how do you do it? When making the transition from nappies to pants, a little guidance can be a great help...

Development during the early years of your child's life is rapid and remarkable. Each milestone reached, from rolling, sitting, and crawling to walking, feeding, and talking, signposts an exciting new stage for your baby and a growing independence. During the early years, the development of skills is often interrelated, with progress in one area leading to advancement in another. Learning to use the potty is a perfect example of how the confluence of several skills brings your child to a point of readiness from which she can learn to exercise control over her bladder and bowel movements – and forego nappies.

While parents look forward to life after nappies, potty training itself is possibly one of the least popular aspects of early years parenting. Whether it's the inevitable accidents, constant vigilance, or the (often) protracted nature of the process, it's easy to see why you might approach the job with a small degree of dread. But as with so many aspects of parenting, forethought and preparation can make the task that much easier.

Throughout this book, the aim is to guide parents through each step of potty training, thinking about how children learn to become clean and

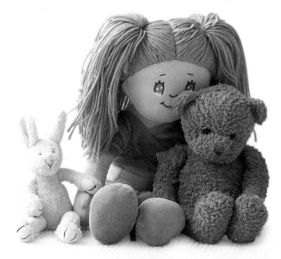

dry in stages and what motivates them to keep at it. Whatever your approach –whether you think it is best to start early and guide your child, or to wait until your little one is more able to take the lead – guidelines, tips, and strategies will help you and your child to negotiate the process as quickly and efficiently as possible.

Chapter One looks at the different approaches to potty training and how trends for starting earlier or later change across generations and cultures. This chapter also explores your child's signs of readiness for potty training, guiding parents on what to look out for and how to pick the best moment to start.

For many children, preparation is the key to successful potty training. Chapter Two runs through essential skills, such as hand-washing and dressing, and highlights the importance of agreeing a toilet-training language within the family so that your little one can quickly express her needs, confident of being understood.

Learning to use the potty is a significant milestone in early childhood.

The third chapter focuses on the moment your child takes the plunge, providing strategies, tips, and advice to help parents negotiate the first few days of going without nappies.

The final chapters look at specific scenarios and concerns, such as coping away from home; dealing with accidents; and managing special situations, including preparing for preschool toilet regimes and coping with medical and special needs. Chapter Six is dedicated to nighttime dryness, the final step in your little one's potty training journey.

Throughout the book, parents are informed and supported, making this a trusty companion for every parent of a potty-training toddler.

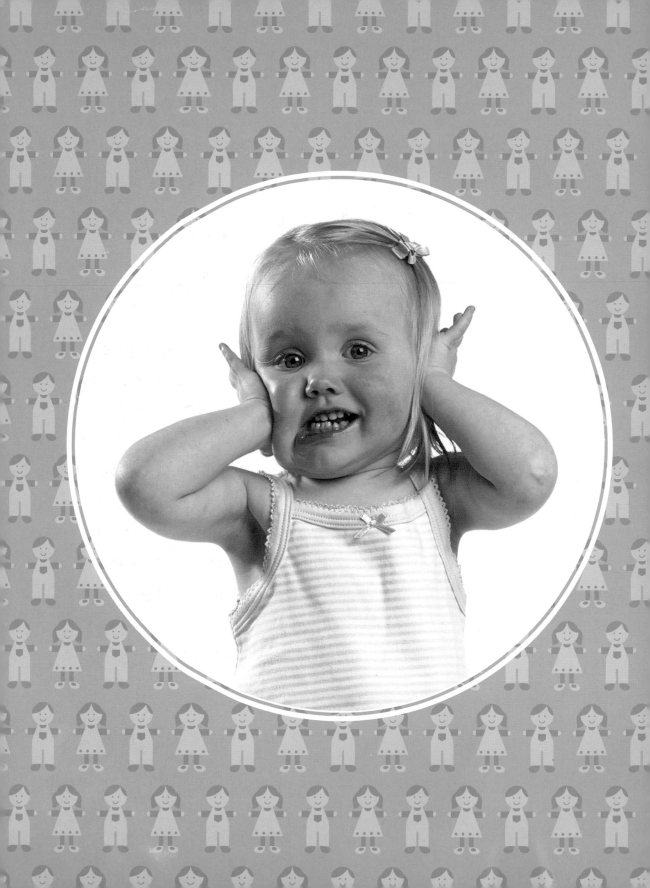

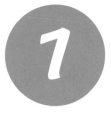

When should we begin?

Potty training your toddler is an exciting parenting milestone as you will soon be saying goodbye to nappies! However, it's also a little daunting, as months of puddles and emergency toilet dashes beckon. So getting the timing right can feel tricky. If you start too soon, will your child resist, or will potty training drag on interminably? And if you leave it too late, will your little one be reluctant to part with her familiar nappies? Understanding how your child develops physically, and watching for signs of emotional readiness, can help you work out the very best time for her to take this significant step, ensuring that potty training is as quick and painless a process as it can be.

How your child develops

The transition from nappies to pants is a significant early years milestone – a clear marker that your little one is growing up. To help potty training run as smoothly as possible, your toddler ideally needs to show readiness in several areas. She should be both physically and emotionally ready, and her brain needs to be developed enough to be able to recognize and act upon signals from the bladder and bowel, which can be the case any time from around 18 through to 36 months.

Gaining control

After months – or years – of changing nappies, you may be eagerly anticipating the switch to the potty or toilet. As well as reducing your workload, waving goodbye to nappies eases the load on your purse, too. However, while you may be keen to introduce the potty at the earliest opportunity, doing so before your little one is completely ready risks prolonging the whole potty-training process. Waiting for the right moment will help ensure that potty training is as smooth and quick a transition as possible.

Your baby isn't born with conscious control over her bowel and bladder, so for the first year or two, a reflex action triggers these to empty automatically when full. At around 18 months of age, nerve pathways

from her bladder and bowel to her brain have developed fully, and at this point she starts to become aware that she is doing a wee or a poo. However, it will be a while yet before she is able to recognize the urge to go and connect this with the need to get to the potty; first, she needs to become familiar with the urge to empty her bladder or bowel, and then she will gradually develop the ability to hold on until she makes it to the potty or toilet. This usually happens at around two and a half years, but can be earlier or later depending on your child. The clearest sign that your child has developed some bladder control is when she manages to stay dry for an extended period of time during the day. Check her nappy regularly to see how dry it is. If you still need to change it fairly frequently, then trying to potty train now is likely to be stressful and impractical. But if she is managing to stay dry for a couple of hours or so, this indicates that she has gained sufficient bladder control to "hold on" long enough to get to a potty.

> *While you may have your own mental time frame for potty training, your child will only truly master it when she is herself ready.*

Your coordinated toddler

As well as having achieved a degree of bladder and bowel control, your child also needs to exhibit other signs of physical readiness before you can be happy that she's ready to start using the potty.

Getting on and off the potty and managing her pants and clothes requires a certain level of coordination for your toddler. This may be tricky for younger children, or those who learned to crawl and walk a bit later than usual. If your child finds these actions frequently challenging, she may get frustrated and upset with her attempts to use the potty, and, in turn, become reluctant to use it at all. On the other hand, if you think that your toddler is emotionally ready to start using the potty (see p12) and she often manages to stay dry for a couple of hours during the day, you might want to let her have a go and be there to help and support her at first with the more challenging aspects.

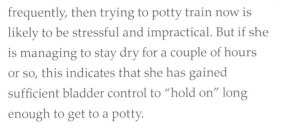

Setting the pace

As with every skill your child masters, potty training is something she will do in her own time at her own pace. While some children are extremely keen and ready to start, taking to the potty almost effortlessly, with few accidents to note along the way, for others it's a somewhat trickier transition. Be reassured, though, that when and how quickly a child becomes potty trained is in no way linked to their intelligence or how quickly they will reach other milestones. So if a child is successful using the potty relatively early, it doesn't then follow that she will learn to talk, write, or read earlier than expected, too.

Older children understandably are more likely to pick up the required skills for potty training quickly as they are more developed. For many, though, it's a fairly slow affair that can take months, and sometimes longer, so try not to get too downhearted by accidents, false starts, or setbacks along the way.

There is evidence of a genetic link with potty training, so asking your parents when you stopped using nappies could be a good indicator of when your child is likely to be ready for the potty. If your child seems ready, this could be the moment to start.

Signs of Readiness

Your toddler is unlikely to tell you that she wants to start using a potty, so you will need to be alert to the signs that she is ready. Many parents start to think about potty training somewhere around their child's second birthday; some toddlers are ready to potty train between 18 and 24 months, although many may need to wait a few months longer. As with all milestones, it's best not to push your child before she is ready. If you can tick several of the points below, your child may well be ready to start:

• Her bowel movements are regular.

• She stays dry for at least two hours in the day, and is usually dry after a daytime nap.

• She is well coordinated, managing to pull trousers up and down and can sit in a squatting position with ease.

• She is aware of when she is doing a wee or poo.

• She shows an interest in what happens when you visit the toilet.

• She is increasingly independent and keen to carry out simple tasks herself.

• She acts on simple requests.

• She is motivated to please you and she mimics your actions.

Emotional readiness

As well as showing signs that she is physically able to cope with potty training, your child needs to be able to understand what is happening when she uses the potty, and be motivated to start potty training.

Look for signs of awareness that she is doing a wee or a poo. She may stop what she is doing, perhaps look at you, or stare fixedly ahead, and may be keen to tell you what she has done. Or she may remove clothes before making a puddle on the floor. This sense of connection with what she is doing is a sign that she is emotionally ready to use a potty.

Showing a willingness to be independent is another good indicator of readiness. If your toddler seems keen to master skills such as doing up zips or putting on clothes and shoes, this shows a level of maturity that means you could start to think about potty training. Of course, not every child is willing to do things for themselves, so if your two and a half year old is happy for you to put on her shoes and pull up her trousers still, you may want to start encouraging her to tackle these things on her own, in preparation for taking on the more challenging task of potty training.

Verbal readiness

By the age of two, your toddler is likely to have a smattering of words and be able to understand many more as she steadily builds up her vocabulary. She may have words for "wee" and "poo" already, which will help her communicate her needs. Being eager to communicate is a big advantage with potty training. Likewise, the ability to follow simple instructions makes potty training easier. For example, being able to understand when you explain what the potty is for, and to act on suggestions such as "Let's look for your potty", will help enormously.

Waiting a little longer

Eager though you may be for your child to be out of nappies, there are times when it's worth waiting a little longer. If your child is younger than 18 months, she's unlikely to have

Your child may be physically ready, but if she isn't mentally ready, potty training may need to wait.

sufficient bowel and bladder control, and if she still shows no awareness of when she wees or poos, or curiosity about what you do in the bathroom, it's worth waiting.

The time when many parents think about potty training, around their child's second birthday, coincides with a period when toddlers are striving for some independence and are keen to exert their own will. This is a perfectly normal stage of development, however, if your child frequently refuses to cooperate, it's probably best to wait until she's feeling a bit more helpful.

It's not uncommon for toddlers still to be in nappies at age three or older; at this age, some might decide themselves that they want to be clean and dry, making the process very smooth

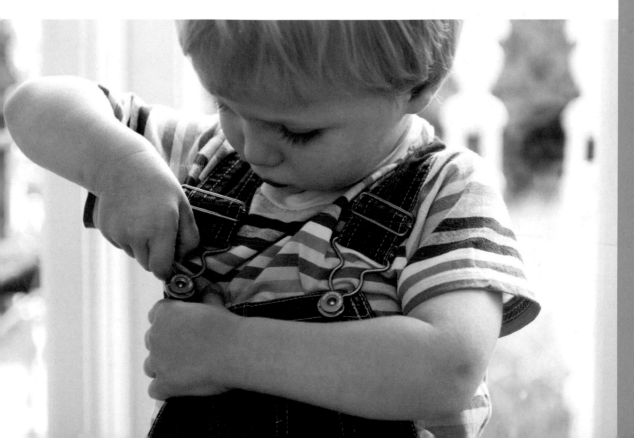

Different approaches

Your approach to potty training – both when to start and how to manage it – often reflects and is influenced by where you live and the accepted norms of your society. There is no right or wrong time or way to potty train, but the age at which your child starts is likely to have a bearing on your level of involvement and how long the process takes.

Did you know?

In parts of India, China, and Africa, potty training sometimes starts at just a few months old. At frequent intervals, or when parents think their child might need a wee or a poo, they simply hold their baby over a toilet, potty, or sometimes a hole in the ground, and make a hissing or whistling noise, similar to that of passing urine.

Deciding when to start

In the West, the received wisdom on potty training is to wait for your child to display signs of maturity and independence before starting (see pp10–13), but in many non-Western cultures, toilet training starts much earlier, often at around a year old, and sometimes even younger. Potty training at a younger age tends to be parent-led as parents watch for signs that their baby is having a bowel movement, or work out when she is likely to need a wee or a poo, for example after a meal or drink, and place her over a toilet or on a potty. Over time, this shows your baby what a potty is for,

although she won't be able to control her bladder and bowel movements and "hold on" for the potty until she's developmentally ready.

Earlier potty training was also more widely practised in the West in previous generations, and in the first half of the twentieth century, toddlers were often started on the potty at 12 to 18 months, creeping up to around 18 months in the 1960s. Part of the motivation to potty train earlier is likely to have come from using cloth nappies, both laborious to clean and less absorbent than disposables today.

Potty training your child when she is older, from 18 months onwards, is a more child-led approach as you wait for signs that your little one is learning to recognize when she needs to empty her bladder or bowel, and you feel confident she will be able

Whatever age your child starts on the potty, she is likely to need help and encouragement at first.

to manage on the potty. Recent studies suggest that the later you wait to potty train your child, the quicker and easier the process is likely to be as all the necessary skills are in place (see p13). If your child seems ready to potty train at 18 months, this could be the time to start. But if the signs aren't quite there, it might be worth holding on a little longer: children who start some time after the age of two are often potty trained in weeks or months; whereas if you start before your child is ready, the whole process could take longer.

Potty training a baby can be a very slow process.

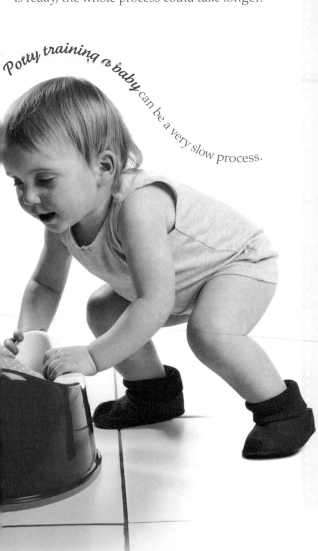

Potty training twins

If you've been kept busy changing two sets of nappies, you are probably highly motivated to potty train your twins as soon as possible. However, as with any child, starting either before they're ready could cause stress and frustration as you find yourself dealing with double the number of puddles and wet pants. Waiting until each twin shows signs of readiness (see p12) will help potty training go smoothly.

It's not unusual for one twin to show an interest earlier than the other. As with all children, twins reach milestones at their own unique pace. While training twins together can seem like the most sensible, time-saving approach, if one clearly is ready earlier, it's best to start with potty training the twin who is ready. Seeing their twin getting on with potty training could be an incentive for the second twin. However, if your second twin still seems reluctant, take care not to turn it into a competition. If she isn't ready to start, she may feel frustrated when her sibling gains attention for something that she isn't able yet to master. Do praise and encourage your potty-training twin, but keep this low-key to avoid tension. Once both twins are in the swing of potty training, a potty each will ensure that both can use a potty at the same time if needed.

Timing it right

While the optimal time to potty train is when your toddler shows signs she is ready, you also need to be in the right frame of mind (see p26), and have enough time set aside to potty train in a calm and relaxed way.

Set time aside

To get off to a good start, and be able to build little by little on what you teach your child, you ideally need a run of a few days where you are with your child and not trying to get a hundred other things done at the same time. Set aside a weekend to devote to the task, and if your little one is in nursery or with their carer all week, it might even be worth taking a Monday or Friday off work so that you can spend three days in a row getting to grips with this new skill. You can then do a handover to her carer who can carry on the good work (see

pp86–9). It will make life easier if you limit outings and social engagements for the first couple of days (or persuade friends to come to you), so that you don't have to cope with potty training while you are out and about.

Whatever the weather

Potty training during the warmer months is ideal as your little one can run around with few, or no, clothes on, making it easier to use the potty as she won't have to remove layers. However, it's best to start when she is ready, so if this happens to be in the winter, don't delay.

Time potty training carefully if you've a new baby on the way

Other things to consider

If your child is undergoing a period of change, for example, starting at a new nursery or childminder's, moving house, or even coping with a bereavement, or parents separating or working away from home more, she may be struggling to take things in her stride. In this case, it's better to take a check on potty training and wait until she's settled back into a predictable routine, when she will be better able to focus.

The arrival of a new baby means your toddler's world is disrupted, so it's not a good time to start potty training.

A new baby on the way

You're expecting a baby and not relishing the thought of two little ones in nappies. If your child is ready to potty train near the start of pregnancy, and you feel up to it, you could try potty training now. The older your child, the quicker the process should be. If, though, potty training is likely to continue after the birth, it's worth waiting, for both your sakes.

Your child is busy getting used to the idea of a new arrival and may be dealing with conflicting emotions. The reality of having to compete with her new brother or sister for mum's attention may make her less cooperative and mean that she is likely to have setbacks until she adjusts and starts to bond with her sibling. While dispensing with one set of nappies may seem tempting, do you want to be dealing with puddles and changes with a newborn in tow?

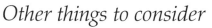

Succumbing to pressure

Resisting outside pressure to potty train can be hard. Grandparents may express surprise that you haven't started yet, reminding you that you were potty trained by your child's age. Or friends' children may be potty training and you're worried that your child seems babyish and is being left behind.

Though hard to resist, try to shut out distractions and focus on what's right for you and your child. A generation ago, before the advent of disposable nappies, early potty training was more in vogue, spurred on largely by a desire to stop washing and drying cloth nappies. Keep in mind that the more ready your child is, the more likely potty training will be speedy and successful.

Potty training is a developmental stage, and as with other skills such as crawling and walking, it's one your child masters with trial and error. Putting pressure on to use the potty before she is ready is likely to result in more accidents and take longer; and the upset caused by frequent wet and soiled pants may make your child resistant.

Being patient and supporting your child when she is ready is likely to produce the best results, and your child will enjoy the boost to her confidence.

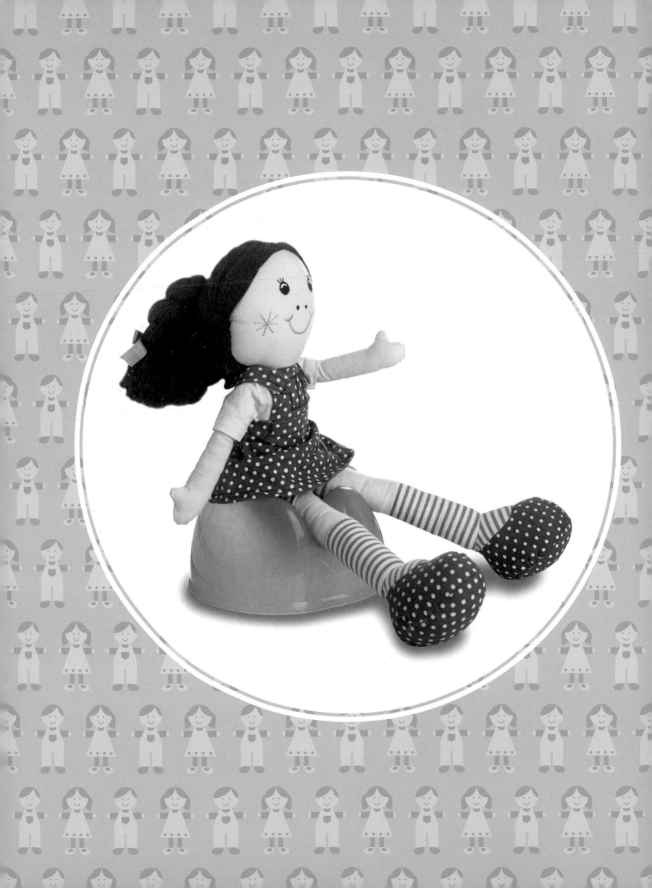

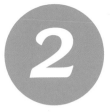

Getting ready

You've noticed that your child is starting to show signs of bladder and bowel control, so what happens next? As with the acquirement of any life skill, putting in a little preparation before you start can pay dividends later on. While some children need scant encouragement to try something new, many appreciate a more gradual introduction. Familiarizing your child with the potty before he is ready to use it, chatting to him about what it's for, and encouraging him to have a go at small, but significant, associated tasks such as dressing and hand-washing will help him to feel ready and motivated to give potty training a try. And make sure you're ready too, practically and mentally, stocking up on everything you will need, and thinking about your approach, strategies, and coping techniques for the weeks or months ahead.

What you need

Aside from a potty or child toilet seat and some pants for your toddler, there's not a great deal you need for potty training. It's worth getting a potty before you intend to start potty training, and have it out from at least 18 months, so your toddler gets used to it being in the house (see p32).

Which potty?

When buying a potty, think about comfort and practicality. Most provide both: made from softly curved, moulded plastic, they are warm and comfortable, easy to wipe clean, and lightweight with a slot for carrying so they can be moved from room to room. Opt for a hard-wearing potty with a broad, sturdy base that is less likely to be knocked over. Some have handy rubber strips on the base for stability.

Potties with a raised back support provide a secure seat. Models with splash guards are available for boys, although they may need reminding to point their willy down! Girls can use these, too, sitting with the splash guard at the back. Some potties have a lid, which is useful for containing smells if you're away from home. Lids are also handy if you need to carry the potty somewhere to empty it, and for car journeys, when the used potty can be placed securely in the boot.

Potty "chairs" have a substantial back support and moulded arms, giving extra support. Larger than a basic potty, these have

Potties come in various shapes, sizes, and colours to suit all possible needs.

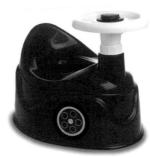

a removable inner potty for easy cleaning. Novelty potties are also available, which can be animal-shaped, musical, or change colour after use, all designed to spark interest; and some are decorated with favourite characters. Letting your toddler personalize his potty with stickers or his name can help him "own" it. Two potties can be handy, for upstairs and downstairs; if you buy identical ones, there's no risk of your toddler favouring one over the other!

Choosing pants

Buying "big boy" or "big girl" pants is a great way to get your little one interested. You could let him choose from the range of fun colours and designs available. Buying two or three sets means you won't be caught short.

It's best to start with normal pants, so your child knows when he has had an accident, but trainer and pull-up pants are also available. Trainer pants are washable cotton pants with a waterproof lining, and pull-up pants are disposable pants made of nappy material that also open at the side, making it easier to check for accidents. See page 37 for the pros and cons of trainer pants and pull-ups.

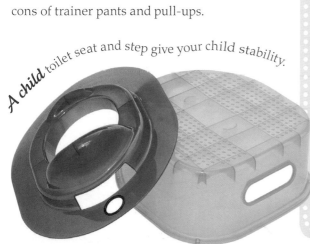

A child toilet seat and step give your child stability.

Other accessories

There are a few other items you may wish to invest in.

• **Child toilet seats** can help the move from potty to toilet, or be used straight away if your toddler is keen. These plastic, sometimes padded, seats go on top of or underneath the existing seat, so your toddler has a secure base and isn't perched precariously on the toilet.

• **A stable plastic step or stool** helps your child to climb onto the toilet seat, gives him somewhere to rest his feet (keeping him stable and focused on going to the loo), and gives him more height at the basin. A step is also useful for boys when they start to stand to wee.

• **Collapsible travel potties** are handy for outings. These come with potty liners, which can be sealed after use and disposed of like a nappy. Some double up as portable toilet seats.

• **"Flushable" wipes** are available, which some parents prefer to toilet roll for cleaning their toddler. However, these don't break down in the same way as toilet roll, and there's growing awareness that they can cause blockages in sewers, so are best binned.

• **Disposable absorbent mats** are handy for damage limitation if your child has an accident on the sofa, in bed, or in his car seat (asleep or awake!).

Preparing your child

Preparing your child gradually for potty training while he is in nappies gives him time to process this information and become familiar with the concept of the potty. One way to help him learn what's expected is to pop a potty in the bathroom a while before you start: you can talk to him about what it's for, and he can sit on it before he actually needs to use it (see p32).

Ready to go!

While the gradual approach works for many, if your toddler is usually keen to dive in and give new things a try, it might be worth waiting until you think he is ready to start potty training, then present a new potty with a flourish, ready for him to use straight away. Or take him with you to buy a potty, then let him try it out when you get home.

Growing independence

For your toddler, an important part of learning to use the potty is having the confidence to try new things on his own. If your child enjoys learning new skills, he may well find potty training fun and exciting. He is at an age when he is likely to be keen to take more control of his world, so may embrace this new challenge. Not all children are raring to go, though. If he's reluctant generally to have a go at certain tasks, such as getting dressed, doing up zips, and washing his hands, give him lots of opportunities to practise these skills to boost his confidence (see pp30–1).

Gently does it

Moving from nappies to the potty is a big step for your toddler, so the more time he has to get accustomed to the idea the better. Aim to strike a balance between encouraging an interest in the potty and not piling on the pressure. You could take him with you to choose a potty, then make sure it's visible in the house and talk to him about what the potty is used for. Be careful not to go overboard, though; you don't want your child to become resistant to the whole idea of the potty when he senses your high expectations.

There's a fine line between encouragement and being over-enthusiastic, so aim to strike a good balance.

Step by step

For your child, going to the toilet is a fairly new concept – even if he has seen you do this many times, he may not have made the connection with himself wetting his nappy or using the potty. It's unrealistic to expect him to sit on a potty and know straight away what

A new potty and new underwear can motivate your child.

to do. Instead, keep the potty in the bathroom, and when you or your partner are using the toilet, talk to your little one about how soon he will be able to use the potty in the same way. Older brothers and sisters, cousins, or potty-trained friends might also be only too delighted to demonstrate how the process works! Taking these steps helps to introduce the idea of using the potty gradually and in a matter of fact way.

The more you can do to help him understand how going to the toilet works, the more normal using the potty will seem to your toddler. Help him to see potty training as a perfectly natural process and an exciting step in his development as he becomes a "big boy", so that he feels secure and loved and has the confidence to give it a go.

When to hold back

If, despite your very best efforts, your toddler continues to show little, or no, interest in sitting on his potty, or any curiosity about what happens when you go to the bathroom, it's probably best to hold off on potty training for the time being and to stop talking about the potty. If he simply isn't ready to think about this yet, even

your very best efforts at making the subject entertaining are likely to fall on deaf ears and could lead to an unhelpful battle of wills.

Never make your toddler sit on the potty if he isn't keen, or get cross with him if he won't try it out. Being forceful or showing your annoyance could make him tearful of the potty and he may start to associate the potty with your cross words, which in turn could set potty training back by several months.

Encouraging your child

Your toddler's world is opening up as his agility, mobility, and language skills develop. He will want to try things for himself more and more, and letting him feel he is in control and can have a go, even if he isn't quite able to manage certain tasks yet, will help to keep him happy and boost his confidence, making the switch from nappies to potty that much easier.

Show him you're enthusiastic when he has a go at something new. He loves to show off a new skill to you, and knowing you're behind him gives him the security to try things out.

Calmly praise him when he succeeds in a task or carries out a simple request such as eating with a fork rather than his fingers. Be alert to his signs of independence and take notice when your child carries out a helpful task such as putting his toys away. When you praise him for his endeavours, he will enjoy your attention and approval and will be motivated when it comes to giving potty training a go.

Don't expect him to do things before he's ready. Try to avoid making unhelpful mental comparisons with friends' children, and remind yourself that all children develop at different rates. If he's really struggling to do something, try to find ways to simplify the task for him so he avoids becoming frustrated and isn't put off trying again another time.

The art of communicating As your toddler's language acquisition increases, your channels of communication grow. Talking face to face, listening patiently when he tries to tell you something, and chatting to him throughout the day will help him to feel confident that he is listened to and understood, all of which will help with potty training.

Toilet talk

Part of the key to successful potty training is ensuring that your toddler is able to communicate his needs and is familiar with the words used for activities to do with the toilet. Agree with your partner on the words you will use as a family, and make sure your child becomes familiar with these words before he starts potty training. This will ensure that he is able to tell you what he needs rather than ending up frustrated when he struggles to make himself understood.

Whether you opt for the ubiquitous "wee" and "poo", or go with "wee wee", "pee", "poop" or "number twos", bear in mind that your child will need to be understood away from home, too, for example at nursery, playgroup, or a childminder's. As your child's vocabulary grows and he starts to form simple sentences, you can teach him to refine how he expresses his need for the toilet by saying something like: "I need the loo please", rather than stating exactly what he needs to do!

Looking at books together

There are plenty of colourful potty-training books on the market that are designed for you and your child to look at together. Familiar and fun characters draw your child in, and simple language is used to introduce the idea of the potty and explain how potty training works and the function of nappies, potties, and toilets. Spend some time reading a book together and leave the book in an accessible place for your child to browse at his leisure.

Make sure that your child is familiar with the words that you as a family use for potty training.

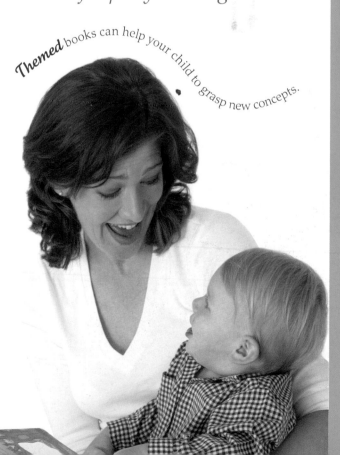

Themed books can help your child to grasp new concepts.

How you're feeling

The time may be just right for your child to start potty training, but are you in the right frame of mind, too? How you set about potty training can have a significant impact on how your child progesses, so before you start, take a moment to think about your approach and whether you need to work generally on your motivational strategies and responses to setbacks.

Your mindset

As with many aspects of your child's development, potty training involves a fair bit of teamwork. Your child will look to you for guidance and instruction on how to use the potty, and, being motivated to please you, will bask in your praise. He will also notice if you are cross or irritated when he has an accident, and this may dent his confidence. It's important, therefore, to examine your mindset before you embark on potty training. While you've had a couple of years already to practise the art of patience – a cornerstone of parenting – potty training is one of those areas where you may be put to the test more than usual.

If it helps, think about potty training not as something that your child needs to get under his belt as swiftly as possible, but rather as a skill, just like walking and talking, that he has to practise in his own good time; at the same time accepting that messy accidents are a rather unfortunate part of the whole process, and not quite as endearing as a tumble on the grass when he was learning to walk. If you know that patience is something you struggle with at times, this may be sorely tried during months of potty training, which is one of the more stressful aspects of parenting during the preschool years. Try to focus on the end goal and remind yourself that getting cross is unlikely to motivate your child, and will most likely prolong the whole process.

Working together

While one parent may be the primary carer, it's important that you and your partner talk about your joint approach so that you can be happy your child won't receive mixed messages, or become worried and confused when one parent reacts in a different way to accidents. Iron out any differences of opinions beforehand and decide together on your potty-training strategy. Agree together to exercise patience, to persevere, and to try to maintain a positive attitude, even when wiping up for the umpteenth time!

Approaching potty training as a family venture ensures a feeling of mutual support.

Be realistic too, though. There's no doubt that there are moments of potty training that are extremely trying, and at times you may feel pushed to your limits, especially when you think your child really should know better. It's not possible, or desirable, to be the perfect parent at all times, and sometimes you won't be able to keep your irritation from showing. While of course it's best not to snap, if you do, apologize afterwards to your child for being a bit cross, and explain that you are just feeling tired with all the wiping up, but you know he will do his best to get to the potty next time.

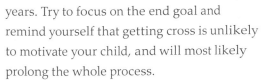

Coping strategies

If at times you feel that potty training is taking forever and that perhaps you've got your approach all wrong, try the following:

• **Remind yourself** that potty training is a learned skill, just like walking. Of course your child has to go to the toilet, but this doesn't mean that using the potty comes easily. As with all skills, making mistakes is part of the learning curve. It's very unlikely that he is having accidents because he is lazy – especially in the early days of potty training when it's all new to him – they happen because it's hard for him to get it right all the time.

• **Aim to be** mutually supportive with your partner. Even if one parent is the main carer, recognize that this is a stressful period and help each other out whenever you can. Have a rota with your partner at the weekends so you each have some time to switch off from potty training.

• **Don't be reluctant** to accept support and practical help from others. You may worry about grandparents or close friends having to deal with your child's potty-training accidents, but if they are willing to help out and give you a break at times, try to relax and accept their offers of help gratefully.

Managing hand-washing

Teaching your child how to wash her hands before she begins potty training will give her one less skill to learn once she does start. Build hand-washing into her daily routine so she gets used to doing it regularly before meals and after playing outside. Guide her through this step-by-step sequence each time, until she knows the routine off by heart.

1. Wet her hands

Show your child how to roll up her sleeves, then turn on the tap, adjusting it to get warm (rather than hot or cold) water, before wetting her hands.

Practice makes perfect

Like all new skills, your toddler may need help at first with hand-washing, but eventually she needs to learn to do this herself. Letting her have a go early on may be messy, but she will learn more quickly. A plastic step will give her the height to concentrate on the task rather than balancing on tiptoes.

2. Wet the soap

Show her how to wet the bar of soap – or use a squirt of liquid soap if a bar is too slippery at first.

3. Lather up

Turn off the tap while she rubs her hands and fingers together to lather up the soap.

4. Rinse well

Show her how to rinse her hands well, checking first the water temperature doesn't need adjusting.

5. Dry thoroughly

Have a small, dry towel to hand, and show her how to dry her hands thoroughly.

Learning new skills

Successful potty training involves more than your toddler simply learning to sit on the potty to do a wee or poo. He also needs to be taught some other practical skills, such as dressing and hand-washing, that will help him to master potty training and ensure that he practises good toilet hygiene.

Managing clothes

If your toddler struggles getting himself dressed, it can be tempting to take over to speed the process up. However, when he starts to use the potty, he will need to be able to undress his bottom half fairly quickly and to pull clothes back up once he's finished. Encourage him to have a go at putting on clothes, building in time if necessary to your morning routine so that he doesn't feel rushed and under pressure. Give him lots of opportunities to practise getting dressed and undressed, but be ready to step in and lend a hand if he needs some help. Avoid clothes with tricky zips or fastenings; instead opt for trousers with elasticated waists that are easy to pull up and down, or dresses and tunics.

Your toddler's life is full of small, but significant, challenges, each one paving the way to independence.

Hand-washing

This essential skill will be an important part of your little one's potty routine. Pages 28–9 have a hand-washing step-by-step that you can look at with your toddler to show him how to manage the hand-washing sequence.

Wiping

Once your toddler begins potty training, he'll start to learn how to wipe himself. Take him to the toilet with you before he starts on the potty and talk to him about what you are doing to help him to understand how and why wiping happens. Show him how to tear sheets off the roll, and how many sheets are needed – young children can get carried away with toilet roll, so it's worth teaching economy. When he starts on the potty, you will probably have to help with wiping for a while as many find this tricky. Little girls need to be taught to wipe from front to back (see p42), and once boys stand to wee, explain how they can shake their willy gently to finish off, rather than wipe.

Helping a reluctant toddler

If your toddler seems unwilling to do even simple tasks, you may feel concerned, especially when it comes to encouraging potty training. This reluctance may simply be an inherent characteristic – perhaps he is anxious about getting things right. If, though, you're concerned that he often holds back, check that you're not stepping in too often to take over, perhaps to do up his coat, or help him solve a puzzle. Your intention is to help, but you may be affecting his confidence to see a task through on his own.

Be wary, too, of having unrealistic expectations. If your toddler feels under pressure to perform, he may become fearful about trying new things in case he fails. Build his confidence with tasks you think he can manage, such as putting vests in a drawer, and praise his efforts. Over time, his confidence should grow.

Try to hold off on potty training until you feel happy that your toddler is willing and motivated. Giving him enough time to practise and consolidate new skills before he starts potty training will help to give him the impetus to succeed when he does begin, and will make it less likely that he will struggle physically or mentally with the process.

Introducing the potty

The first step in potty training is introducing the potty. Having a potty in the house from at least 18 months old means your toddler gets used to seeing it, and you can talk to him about what it's for and how he can use it when he's a bit older – unless of course he's keen to start straight away!

Where to put the potty

The most logical place for the potty is in the bathroom. Keeping it here means that your toddler will start to make the connection between the toilet and his potty. However, if he moves the potty around the house, try to resist the urge to stop him or to return it to the bathroom. Taking ownership of the potty is a healthy sign that he is interested and motivated, and deciding where to put it gives him a sense of control and independence that will be advantageous when he starts to use the potty.

Just like you

You are your child's first teacher and he loves to watch and imitate what you do. Being relaxed about using the toilet while he is with you, and talking to him about what is happening, is a great help as you build up to potty training. He will make associations and develop a good understanding of what's happening, and is also likely to be motivated to be like you.

Trying out the potty

It's a good idea to encourage your child to sit on the potty with his clothes on at first so he gets used to the feel of it and has plenty of time to practise getting on and off – before he needs to do this when he's in a hurry. Don't insist, though, if he's reluctant at first, as this could create negative feelings towards his

Playing with his potty signals your toddler's interest.

potty. He may simply play with his potty at first, putting toys on and taking them off and exploring the look and feel of it, before he progresses to sitting on the potty.

Once he is used to sitting on the potty with his clothes on, you could suggest he tries this without his nappy, perhaps after an evening bath or between nappy changes. If he does a wee or a poo while sitting on the potty without his nappy, offer him gentle praise, but don't go overboard as he may feel pressure to perform like this each time he sits on it – it was most likely just good timing the first time rather than an intentional act. Encourage him to sit on his potty daily, and don't limit the amount of time he sits there if he enjoys it – the more time he spends on it now, the more receptive he is likely to be to the idea of using it properly later on.

In the days before you start potty training, encourage your toddler to sit on the potty more than usual. Time these moments for when he's likely to do a wee or a poo, for example after a drink or a nap. Even if he sits on it for just a few moments each time, he will be increasing his familiarity with the potty.

Taking time

There's no magical timetable for when potty training should start and how long it will take – it really is down to your child's readiness and motivation. So if you think your little one is physically ready, but he still pays scant attention to the potty, try to be patient and eventually you will find his interest grows. The box, right, has some fun ideas to make potty training seem more enticing.

Make it fun

If your little one consistently ignores the potty or only sits on it for a moment, there are plenty of fun ways to ignite his interest. The more he connects sitting on the potty with happy, contented moments, the more relaxed he'll be when he uses it.

• **Engage him** in potty role play. Place his favourite teddy on the potty so that he can play "mummy" or "daddy", telling teddy how to use it.

• **Put a few toys** next to the potty for him to play with while he sits there, or a couple of books for him to leaf through.

• **Suggest he sits** on the potty while you read a favourite story book. Look at the pictures together and chat about the book.

• **Get an older sibling or friend** who he looks up to to show him how to use the toilet and potty. Toddlers are fascinated by older children and are often keen to imitate them.

• **Look at a colourful, fun book** about potties together.

• **Suggest he sits** on the potty while you watch a cartoon together.

• **Take him shopping** to buy some "big boy" pants. Explain what these are for, and that he can wear his new pants when he is ready.

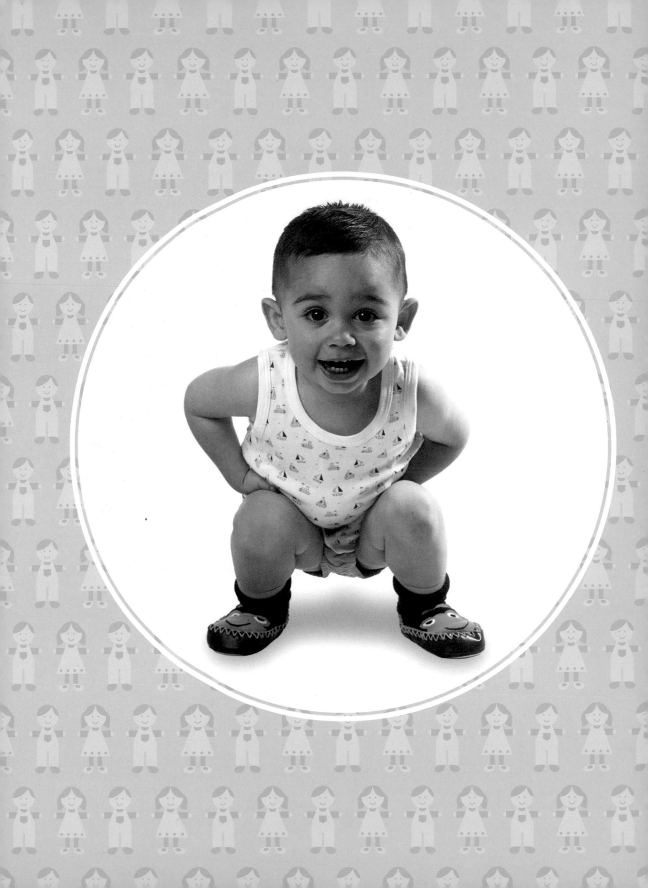

3

Nappy off!

Your toddler is ready, you've spent time preparing him, and now it's time to start potty training! The first week or so out of nappies can be quite a learning curve for both of you, so allowing yourselves some uninterrupted time and space to muddle through these first few important days can make all the difference. Your toddler will, understandably, need a bit of guidance and quite a lot of support as he tackles this new skill. Being aware of the ways in which you can help him practically, as well as thinking about how you can keep him feeling motivated and emotionally supported, will ensure that he doesn't feel daunted and will give him the confidence boost he needs to give potty training his very best shot.

First nappy-free days

You've prepared your child for potty training, cleared your diary for the next couple of days, and now the time feels right to try putting her in pants for the first time. Exciting though this moment is for you, try to keep it low-key so your child doesn't sense your expectation. Being matter of fact and relaxed, encouraging and praising your child along the way, will help potty training go as smoothly as possible.

Your role

Your toddler may be ready to start using the potty, but this doesn't mean that she will be able to cope completely on her own. At first she will probably need prompting and reminding when you think she needs the loo, as well as help with clothes and wiping herself.

It's important that you feel prepared, too. Decide on your approach when you start. Will you lead the way, actively sitting your child on the potty at regular intervals so that she gets used to this? Or would you prefer for her to lead the way – letting her know the potty is there and what it's for, and telling her she can sit on it when she chooses to, then leaving her to decide when she wants to use it? Whichever approach you choose, be prepared to be a bit flexible. If your toddler resists sitting on the potty when you ask her to, you might need to give her a bit more autonomy, so she feels she has some control; alternatively, if once you've introduced the potty and you're confident she is ready to start, but time passes without her asking to use it, you might need to intervene a little and introduce some "potty time" – perhaps she just needs a little nudge.

Well prepared

Make sure you have everything you need to hand when your child starts to use the potty. This includes a good supply of pants as there are bound to be accidents along the way. Reward systems are usually more appropriate later on when initial enthusiasm wanes and some encouragement to keep going is needed. However, you might want to give some thought now as to whether you will use an incentive if you think it would be helpful, and what this might be (see p45).

Getting started

On day one of potty training, tell your toddler that she won't be wearing her nappy today and that instead she will wear "big girl" pants (or trainer or pull-up pants; see box, right). If she wants to try to pull these up herself, let her go ahead so that she feels independent, reassuring her you're there to help if needed.

Tell her to try to let you know when she needs a wee or a poo so that you can quickly fetch her potty. You might want to have more than one potty in the house, perhaps one upstairs and one downstairs, so that there's always one reassuringly close by.

> *Your toddler's first attempts at using the potty may need refining. Be ready to step in and help when needed.*

Bear in mind that as nappies are so highly absorbent, your toddler may have little idea to begin with that wee actually comes out of her body. The first time she realizes this may be when it's trickling down her leg! If the weather permits, setting up some activities outside on the first couple of days can remove much of the stress of clear ups. If you have a garden, take the potty outside, too, and tell your little one it's there if she needs a wee.

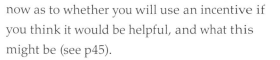

Pants or pull-ups?

If you don't feel ready to go cold turkey and dispense with nappies altogether, putting your toddler in pull-up or trainer pants (see p21) initially, until she becomes more comfortable using the potty, can be a way to make the process more gradual.

Pull-up or trainer pants are styled like normal pants, so your toddler can pull them up and down as she would pants, but they absorb accidents, especially pull-ups, which are made of nappy material, so your toddler is eased gently into potty training. The disadvantage is that your toddler is less likely to sense when she is wet, so it could take her longer to make the connection between doing a wee and using the potty. And if it feels as though she is still wearing a nappy, she may feel she doesn't need to bother with the potty after all.

You might also want to think about whether to use both pants and pull-up nappies for a while, perhaps sticking to pants at home, but wearing a pair of pull-ups when you're out shopping or on a day trip. The danger is this risks confusing your child and could slow her progress, as well as be demotivating.

Help and encouragement

Be prepared to be extra vigilant so you can spot the signs when your child needs the loo. Your on-the-go toddler is often so distracted by other activities, that she may find it hard to break off from what she is doing to go and use the potty; and in the early days of potty training, she may not actually recognize the sensation of needing the loo for what it is. Wriggling, suddenly hopping and jumping about, squeezing her legs together, holding herself, or not being able to concentrate on an activity, are all classic signs that your toddler needs a wee or a poo, so step in and gently take her to the potty.

Give her plenty of praise in these early days when she uses the potty, or even just tries to get to it. If she has an accident, don't make a big fuss. Just wipe up and change her matter of factly, telling her not to worry and that she can try to get to the potty next time.

Encourage her to tell you when she is wet or soiled so that you can change her promptly into clean, dry clothes, which in turn will help to develop her awareness of when she has done a wee or a poo.

It's early days, and accidents are part and parcel of the process, so try to take these in your stride.

What to expect

It's best to accept that accidents are a very normal part of potty training, and actually help your child to connect the sensation of needing to go to the loo with the action of going, so that next time she is more likely to make it to the potty.

Young children wee around every two hours or so, around four to eight times during the day, and can have a bowel movement one to two times a day. Your toddler is unlikely to make it to the potty reliably each time when she starts potty training, and in the first few

Potty hygiene

It's easy to tip your child's wee down the toilet bowl and give the potty a quick wipe over. Cleaning out a poo can be a bit messier. One trick is to pop a piece of toilet roll in the potty if your toddler indicates she needs a poo, then simply lift this out and flush it down the loo and give the potty a quick wipe afterwards. Some parents are shocked when their child touches their poo. As unwelcome as this is, your toddler is simply fascinated by what has come out of her body, and, as with everything she encounters, she is keen to explore! Avoid sounding disgusted. Just tell her matter of factly that it's better not to play with her poo, then remove the potty and poo and wash her hands thoroughly.

days, she may have as many as several accidents a day. As with learning any skill, making mistakes allows your child to work out why something has happened, and what she can do next time to avoid it happening again. Frustrating though this is, don't get cross or make a fuss. Chapter Five has plenty of tips on how best to deal with accidents, as well as reassurance that these will eventually pass.

Straight to the toilet?

Some parents decide to bypass the potty altogether and move straight to the toilet if they think their child is ready for this. While this could work well for some, there are a few advantages of the potty over the toilet during

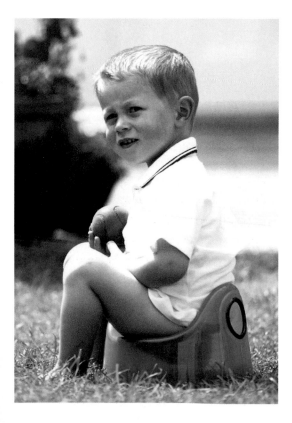

Helpful tips
You can help
your child by being alert to the signs that she needs the loo, such as wriggling or hopping up and down. As well as being watchful, help her by:
• dressing her in easily managed clothes, such as trousers with elasticated waists.
• not giving up at the first hurdle. Try to avoid going back to nappies if you can.
• Briefing a regular carer on your approach.

the first few months that it's worth taking into account. The most obvious advantage is that the potty is transportable, so can be moved from room to room as your toddler moves around, and, in the early days, placed promptly underneath her when she needs it. It's also easy to take on car journeys, visits to family, and on days out.

For most young children, a potty is less daunting at first than the big toilet, which many toddlers are fearful of (see p49). If your child takes a little time to get used to new things, a potty is probably a gentler introduction to toilet training. And from a practical point of view, the position your little one adopts while squatting on a potty makes it easier for her to do a poo.

Ultimately, though, it's down to what's best for you and your child, and your child's personality. If she seems keen to use the toilet, a child toilet seat (see p21) can help her to use it comfortably, and this saves you getting her used to a toilet later on.

Staying clean and dry

You've waited for the right moment and potty training is underway. For your toddler, though, staying clean and dry isn't something she can achieve immediately – it usually takes time.

The three stages of potty training

Becoming aware that she has done a wee or a poo is the first step towards being clean and dry. You can help her to start developing this awareness by prompting her to sit on the potty at opportune moments, such as after a meal or when she wakes after a nap. Gradually, she will start to connect sitting on the potty with the act of relieving herself.

Your toddler starts to recognize the sensation of needing to empty her bladder and bowel, and lets you know when she wants to use her potty. She still hasn't learned to hold on for any length of time, though, so when she says she wants to use her potty, she will need it quickly – be prepared to act swiftly!

How long does it take?

There's no definitive timetable for how long potty training takes. It is thought that girls tend to grasp the basics more quickly than boys (see p43), but generally your toddler sets the pace. Of course, some children get the gist of potty training in no time at all and are more or less home and dry within a week. For most, though, you can expect the process to take several months, and sometimes even longer.

Managing to stay dry takes plenty of practice and is something that happens gradually in stages (see above), so your little one needs to be given ample time to gain experience and to try out her potty in a variety of situations before you can be confident that she has truly mastered the ability to stay dry. Understanding what happens in each stage of potty training will enable you to offer the appropriate level of support for whichever stage your child is at, bolstering her confidence along the way.

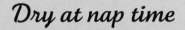

Which comes first?

The order in which children achieve bladder and bowel control can vary, but it's quite common for bowel control to come first. A healthy diet helps regular bowel patterns to develop. It's also usually physically easier to hold a bowel movement long enough to get to a potty, whereas holding a wee can be more challenging.

As your toddler's bladder and bowel muscles get stronger, and her bladder capacity increases, she will be better able to hold on, allowing you time to fetch her potty, or for her to reach it and get undressed. Depending on her age, it will probably take at least a couple of months before she reaches this stage.

Dry at nap time

You may wonder if you should pop a nappy on for daytime naps, or simply hope for the best. While putting a nappy on might seem to make perfect sense – after all, you don't expect her to stay dry when she's asleep at night – daytime naps are usually no more than a couple of hours, a length of time your toddler can probably stay dry for now. Putting a nappy on her for naps could be confusing, as well as undermine the work she has been doing to stay dry.

To help avoid accidents during daytime naps, try putting your toddler on the potty before she settles down to sleep. Placing a protective plastic covering under her sheet will make cleaning up easier if she does have an accident during naptime. When you're out with the buggy or in the car, keep a towel or absorbent mat handy so you can slip this under her if she falls asleep in transit.

As with all accidents, don't make a fuss or show annoyance if your toddler wets herself during a nap. In fact, this is especially important for naptime accidents as staying dry while asleep is not something she has control over (see pp76–7). Change clothes and bedding without a fuss, and reassure her that over time she will manage to stay dry.

Boys and girls

While most potty-training advice applies in equal measure to boys and girls, there are a few gender-specific points that it's worth being aware of, and which may help you avoid certain problems and pitfalls.

Girls only

Teach your little girl to sit well back on the potty to avoid wee splashing out and wetting her pants, clothes, and shoes. Encourage her, too, to pull her pants right down to her ankles once she has sat down so these are well out of the way, or, if she prefers, take them off completely. If she needs to do a wee when outside in the garden or at the park, it can be tricky for her to hold a squatting position that avoids getting her pants and clothes wet, so be ready to support her.

Learning to wipe their bottom is something that many toddlers take a while to master, and often it can be easier and less daunting for your child if you help her out with this particular task in the early stages of potty training. However, if your little girl is keen to do this for herself, she needs to learn to wipe carefully to avoid bacteria passing from the anus to the vagina, which could lead to a urinary tract infection (see p93). Show her how to wipe from the front to the back, even if she has only done a wee, and give her regular reminders to do this so she gets in the habit. You can suggest that you have a quick check when she has finished to ensure she is clean and dry, giving her one last wipe if necessary.

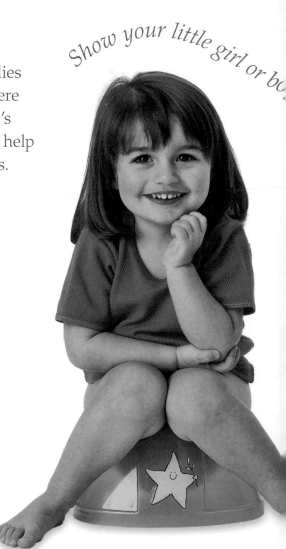

Show your little girl or bo[y]

Boys only

It's usually easier for boys to start off using the potty to wee rather than standing and weeing directly into the toilet, which involves a few additional skills and could be a little daunting. A potty with a splashback is ideal for a boy, but you may still need to remind him to point his willy downwards, or gently do this for him at first, to avoid a sudden spray! Often toddlers have a bowel movement at the same

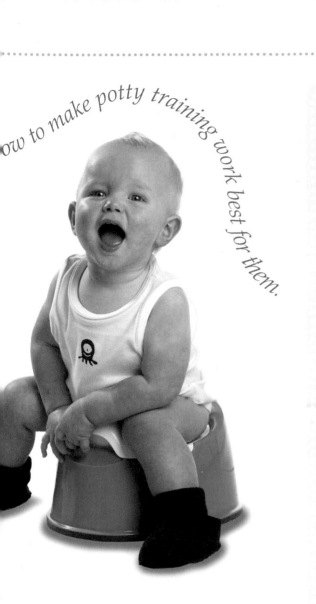

ow to make potty training work best for them.

Do girls potty train faster than boys?

It does seem to be the case that, usually, girls master potty train a few months earlier than boys. So what are the reasons behind this? While there is no one definitive reason why boys tend to be a little bit slower to reach this milestone, there are several possible contributory factors.

Some experts point out that girls often socialize and develop language skills earlier than boys, and this helps them to understand the potty-training process sooner, and means that they may be more able than boys to communicate their needs. In addition, boys tend to be on the go for much of the time, so spending focused time sitting down on the potty is likely to be a less appealing activity.

Often, mums are the primary carer so are providing a constant role model for their little girls; while little boys might not be very aware of anatomical differences at this age, they may instinctively relate to dad more than to mum. And, of course, for boys, having a choice of whether to sit or stand to do a wee gives them one more thing to think about, which could manage simply to confuse them.

time as a wee, so until your little boy can feel the difference between a bowel and a bladder movement, this is an additional reason to start him off sitting on the potty rather than standing at the toilet. When he does begin to stand at the toilet, there are plenty of tips to help him aim well (see p49).

As with girls, your little boy will probably be happy for you to wipe his bottom for the time being, or to finish off if he's keen to have a go at wiping himself.

Supporting your child

The first few weeks out of nappies can be a trying time, but it's important to avoid showing frustration and be realistic about what your child will achieve now, and over the coming months. Be encouraged, though, that there is plenty you can do to help her along the way.

Being patient and positive

Try to keep emotion out of potty training. Young children are keen barometers of mood, so if she senses that you are extremely eager for her to succeed, she may feel under pressure, which could in turn inhibit her and put her off trying. Do praise her when she uses the potty, or even tells you she needs it but doesn't quite make it, but be matter of fact: you can give her a hug, tell her well done, and let her know how clever she is, but don't go over the top. The best way to encourage your child is to adopt a patient and positive attitude, so she feels supported, no matter how many accidents she has along the way.

In the early days of potty training, expect to offer plenty of practical support.

Be realistic about how much she can cope with at first. Getting to grips with using the potty is quite a challenge for many toddlers; not only are they learning to recognize when they need to go, but they also have to get to the potty on time, manage their clothes and new pants, get clean and dressed afterwards, and wash their hands. Stay close by so you can lend

a hand: look out for signs she needs the potty and bring it to her, help her pull clothes up and down, and help with wiping. She will grow more confident with these skills over time as she becomes familiar with the routine, but lending a hand in the early stages helps to avoid her being overwhelmed and consequently put off.

Learn to take accidents in your stride (see pp60–3). Of course these can be unpleasant,

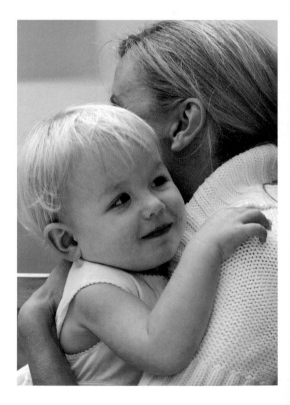

but it's really important that your toddler isn't made to feel bad for not getting to the potty. Clean up calmly and without a fuss, help her get changed quickly so she's not stuck for long in wet clothes, and simply say "Oh dear, don't worry, next time you can try to use the potty."

What to avoid

Your child is learning a new set of skills, which can be stressful, and she's also at an age when she is striving for independence, so pressure from you to do something can result in power struggles. Knowing what to avoid can help to smooth the path.

Parents love to discuss their child's progress, and parents of other toddlers are the perfect audience for your potty-training woes as mutual interest is guaranteed. However, discussing your child's progress, or lack of, in front of her risks her feeling a sense of failure, and could make potty training feel like an onerous task. Tempting though it is, steer clear of the subject.

Avoid pressure. Going to the loo is a natural act that isn't done on demand. If your child feels expected to perform, this could make her anxious, leading to more accidents or her holding back bowel movements, which in a worst-case scenario could cause constipation (see pp92–3).

Never punish your toddler for not making it to the potty, even if you feel she's being wilful. Showing anger is counterproductive: it can ignite the situation and your toddler will develop negative associations with the potty, which is likely to prolong the process. Likewise, never make her sit on the potty until she's done something. This could feel like a punishment and she may start to fear or resent the potty.

Using rewards

There is debate about the worth of using a reward system for potty success. Some see it as a handy aid when initial enthusiasm wears off, while others think that giving rewards can set a precedent, and that using them adds to the sense of failure when "targets" aren't met.

Your child may respond to subtle forms of encouragement, so it's worth trying these before setting up a more tangible reward. Consistent praise can work wonders, and if you're lucky, that may be all that is needed. Or tap into your child's desire to do things for herself, showing her how to tear off toilet roll, and even how to tip the potty contents down the toilet bowl (but don't be cross if she misses!).

For other toddlers, though, a reward system may be beneficial. Some respond brilliantly to a simple star chart. Let her choose a star and stick it on her chart when she uses the potty. Tell her a treat is in store after a certain number of stars. Phoning grandparents as a reward can engender a sense of achievement, too. Rewards need to be given close to the act, as your child won't connect a reward at the end of the day with something she did in the morning. Be clear about what the reward is, so she can't ask for something else, and keep rewards small, especially if offering an edible treat!

Your child's motivation

Parental motivation for potty training is clear, but for success you need to ensure that your child is motivated, too. Unlike other skills, such as crawling, your child may not see an obvious gain, so you need to think about what's in it for her, and try to steer her to recognize the advantages of being able to use the potty. As well as outward motivators, such as rewards, work on inner motivation, for example by increasing her confidence generally, and encouraging her desire to be "all grown up".

In the routine

If your child is clear about what's expected of her, she's more likely to feel she can master each step and will get satisfaction from the routine. Talk her through the sequence of events – getting to the potty, wiping, eventually flushing, and washing hands.

What motivates her?

Your child may be physically able to master a new skill, but to want to have a go, she needs inner motivation. With potty training, think about her personality and age: what's likely to make her tick? For a two year old, this may be being like a big sibling, or you, her ultimate role model. For a child who likes to please, or a three year old in need of renewed motivation, a tangible reward may be the thing.

Making rewards work

If you're using rewards, try tailoring these to your child's age. For younger children, a simple sticker can work wonders, or a star chart displayed prominently so family can praise her achievements. Give stars straight after using the potty. An older child may need another layer to a reward, with stars exchanged for an end-of-week treat, such as a playground trip, comic, or small edible treat.

Stepping in

Learning any new skill is trial and error for your little one. As a parent, your job is to learn when to hold back and let her have a go, but also to spot when she's not coping well and step in before frustration builds – and motivation is lost.

A sense of achievement

Potty training is essentially about mastering a series of small challenges. As each one is met, your child feels satisfaction and continued motivation. Problems in one area can throw her, so make sure she's coping with hand-washing, wiping, and dressing so her confidence isn't dented.

Using the toilet

If your toddler has been using the potty successfully, you might feel it's time to encourage her to give the toilet a try, or she may be keen to do this herself. Or perhaps she expressed an interest in using the toilet early on. Whenever she starts to use the toilet, there are a few things you can do to ensure that it's comfortable and easy for her to manage. If she's due to start preschool or nursery soon, learning to use the toilet will be especially helpful.

What to consider

The toilet bowl can seem scarily big for a young toddler. While some children can have exaggerated fears about falling down the loo (see box, opposite), the fear of slipping isn't entirely unwarranted and there are accessories you can use to help prevent this, such as a child toilet seat and a plastic step (see p21), which make sitting on the toilet a comfortable, secure, and relaxing

A natural transition

Your little one may feel attached to her potty, and need help to see the toilet as the next step. Encourage her to sit on the seat when she doesn't need a wee or a poo so she gets used to being higher up. Reading her a story while she sits there will help her relax. Show her too that this is where her potty contents go so it makes sense to her to use it.

experience for your child. Make sure the child seat is securely attached, otherwise a wobbly toilet seat attachment could prove tricky to sit on and be an additional worry for your child. As well as helping your toddler to get onto the toilet, a plastic step offers a solid base for her to rest her feet on, keeping her steady and secure: this is crucial as it helps her to relax and concentrate on what's she doing. A step can also be useful when boys start to wee standing up, giving them that little bit of extra height if they need it.

Keep the toilet roll within easy reach, and show your toddler how to flush once she has finished and move the step over to the basin to stand on while she washes her hands.

Standing to wee

Little boys often prefer to sit down on the toilet to wee at first, just as they did with the potty. At some point, though (and when he can differentiate between doing a wee and a poo), it's a good idea to teach your child to stand up to do a wee, like Daddy or other big boys do. Before your little one starts, make sure he knows to put the toilet seat up, and back down again once he has finished, and, importantly, ensure that the seat is stable when it's upright so that he doesn't get a shock, or even hurt, if it falls down.

If your little boy is resistant to standing, don't force the issue. He will stand when he is ready to do so.

Getting his wee accurately into the toilet bowl can be quite a skill, so be prepared for plenty of toilet and floor wiping while he practises. In the meantime, there are ways to help him perfect his aim. Try floating a piece of toilet paper in the bowl and get him to soak it; or, for additional fun, pop a ping-pong ball in the loo as target practice! Avoid getting cross if he misses repeatedly; just gently remind him to try to aim for the bottom of the bowl when he goes to the loo.

Overcoming toilet fears

It may seem odd to us, but some toddlers have specific, and to them very real, fears of the toilet, which can put them off using it.

Some children worry that they will fall into the toilet, and may even fear being sucked away with the flush. Some dislike seeing their poo flushed away, as they view this as part of their body. (This may explain why some toddlers prefer to continue with nappies for poos.) Avoid being dismissive. Acclimatize your toddler to the toilet gradually. If she's nervous about sitting on it, get her to practise with the lid down, then to sit on the seat with her clothes on before using it properly. You could consider replacing the loo seat with an integrated child/adult seat, in which the child seat fits securely on top of the adult seat, always ready for your little one to use.

If your toddler doesn't like the noise of the flush, or seeing the contents washed away, resist telling her this is silly. Get her used to the flush slowly. At first, let her leave the bathroom, then flush the loo yourself. Next suggest she stands by the door while you flush. Progress in this way until she watches the contents of the loo flush away, and then is confident to try for herself.

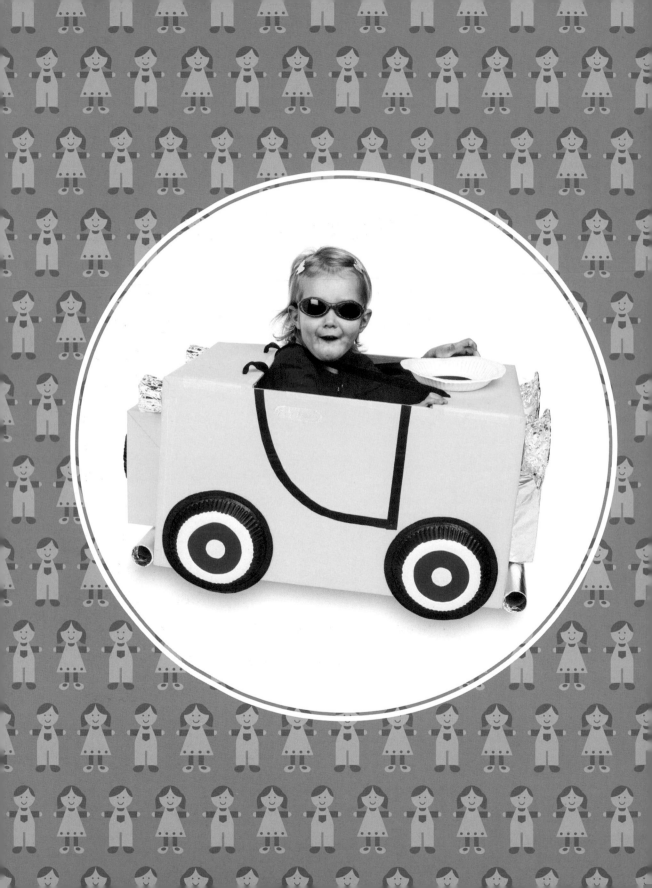

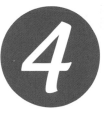

Out and about

Potty training is underway, and there's no doubt that this adds a whole new dimension to excursions. While you may wish to stay on safe turf for the first few days, at some point you will need to take the plunge and venture out. You may feel the need to take a deep breath the first time you leave the safe confines of your home and the on-tap toilet facilities! Of course, there are bound to be hairy moments, but you may well be surprised at just how quickly you and your toddler adapt to coping with her toilet needs away from home. Before long, you'll have route planning and bag packing down to a fine art, and managing toilet stops while out and about will eventually become second nature.

What to think about

In the early stages of potty training, it may seem easiest simply to avoid too many trips out with your toddler. However, while of course accidents can and will happen, with planning and preparation, outings can be managed without too much hassle, giving you both more confidence.

A break from routine

If your toddler is starting to develop a potty-training routine at home, getting used to where the potty is and maybe using it at regular intervals, being away from home could throw him off kilter. Be aware that he is likely to be more distracted when out and may not pay attention to toilet cues, so be extra vigilant to signs that he needs the toilet.

Stepping out

Leaving the house, and the security of having easy access to a potty and toilet, with your potty-training toddler can feel like a brave step, especially if you have to navigate a long trip on the motorway, or visit a house-proud friend! You may be tempted to pop a nappy on for shopping trips, long car journeys, and when visiting other locations where you think you might be caught short. However, it's best to avoid doing this if you possibly can, so that your child doesn't receive mixed messages. He is learning to hold on for the toilet, so using nappies may confuse him and undermine his achievements thus far. If you do go down this route, make sure your child knows these are special "going out pants", and change him into normal pants as soon as you get home.

You will soon get the hang of potty training away from home.

If you can be flexible about what time you leave the house, it can be worth waiting until just after your toddler has used the potty, although this isn't always entirely reliable as there will be days when he decides he needs his potty more frequently. When he is older, you can ask him to visit the bathroom before you go out to see if he needs to do a wee. However, it's extremely hard and confusing for him to respond to this request early on in the potty training process, when he is still trying to get the hang of when exactly he needs the toilet.

Learning to go without a nappy away from home will give your little one a great confidence boost.

Taking the potty with you on outings can work well in the early stages of potty training. It's usually possible to find a discreet spot to use it – if there's no public toilet handy, you can use the potty in the park, or even in the car park or down a quiet side street. If you prefer not to carry a bulky potty around, a collapsible travel potty (see p21) is handy for outings. These are lightweight and have leak-proof absorbent liners that can be disposed of easily. As your child gets older, you may find he becomes less keen to use his potty in open places. If he has started using the toilet at home, it makes sense to get him used to using public toilets in different locations (see p55). Some travel potties double up as portable toilet seats so are ideal for use on public toilets.

What to pack

It's best to expect that your child will need the toilet at some point while you're out of the house and to be well prepared for this eventuality, rather than just hoping for the best, in which case you may find your trip is cut short when you have to return home prematurely to change his clothes. So don't pack away the changing bag just yet. As well as a potty, the following items are helpful:

• **Disposable wipes** can be a godsend away from home, ensuring that you can clean up any major messes, as well as wipe out the potty after use.

• **A couple of plastic bags** are handy, using one for used wipes, and one for wet and soiled clothes.

• **At least one change of clothes**. If you're out for more than a couple of hours, you might need to change your toddler's clothes more than once.

• **A plastic bag and/or towel** to protect the fabric on the buggy seat if your toddler is likely to be spending much time in his buggy.

• **A bottle of water** is handy for cleaning hands after using the potty.

At the shops

If you make regular trips to the supermarket or shopping centre, these could feel especially challenging during potty training. The secret to a successful shopping outing with your potty-training toddler is to think ahead. Consider where you're going and how long you are likely to be out, so that you can plan toilet stops and pack items to deal with any mishaps.

Making it work

Before you set off, make a mental note of the toilet facilities at your destination if you're not taking a potty with you. Does the supermarket you're visiting have customer loos, and where are the toilets located in the four-storey shopping centre? When you arrive at your destination, it's worth checking out the toilets before you do anything else. As well as locating them, this could mean that your toddler feels more comfortable using them later on if he needs the loo in a hurry.

> ### Plan ahead for shopping trips so you and your toddler aren't caught out.

When nature calls

You've come prepared (see box, p53), but it's easy to panic when your child informs you he needs the loo now! Try to react calmly and swiftly.

Quickly assess your options. If you have a potty with you, find the nearest secluded place to use this. If you are out without the potty, ask shop staff for the nearest loo, or pop into a café or restaurant, who will usually understand your plight and allow you to use their facilities. If you're faced with a queue for a public loo, don't be hesitant to ask if you can jump the queue, explaining that your little one can't hold on for long – most people will be more than happy for you to go in front of them. And in shops or establishments without a public toilet, you can always ask if there is a staff loo that you could use.

In the worst-case scenario of your toddler wetting or soiling himself, avoid showing anger or annoyance. Deal with your child calmly and sympathetically – he may feel extra sensitive having an accident away from home, so bear this in mind. Find the nearest loo, or return to the car if you are driving, then get him cleaned up and into dry clothes. Tell him not to worry, that accidents happen, and he can try to remember to let you know next time that he needs a wee or a poo, then don't mention it again.

Using public toilets

Even if your child is getting used to going on the toilet at home, he may worry about using public toilets, which can feel less private, are often smelly and uninviting, and can have alarmingly noisy hand dryers! Some older children may even try to hold on until they get home. However, holding back on going to the loo can cause discomfort and could even lead to constipation (see pp92–3), so isn't advisable. Getting your child accustomed to using a

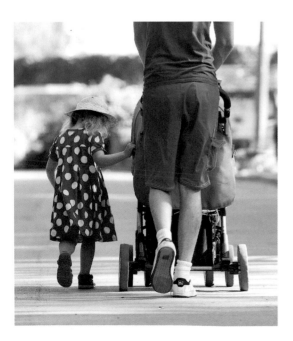

Cutting the stress

While you don't want to be marooned at home just because you're potty training, it's not a bad idea to avoid over-long shopping trips that could be challenging. Now could be a good time to set up an online shopping account, or, if possible, save supermarket trips for times when one partner can look after your child while the other one shops.

variety of public loos will help him overcome any reluctance and increase his confidence. Help him feel secure by staying with him in the cubicle, helping with the lock, cleaning the seat if necessary (a bag of wipes can be handy), and supporting him on the seat. When he's finished, help him with wiping and getting dressed and show him how the flush works.

No-one tends to bat an eye when mums take their little boys into the women's toilets in shopping centres, or at motorway facilities. However, it can be more awkward for dads to take their young daughter into the men's toilets, where open urinals make for a different environment. If the men's toilets have cubicles, one option is for dad to carry his daughter briskly through to a cubicle. Alternatively, well-equipped shopping centres, stores, and motorway services have family, or parent and child, rooms, which are a perfect solution for dads and daughters. Or, if it's not in use, a quick dash into the disabled loo is usually okay if the need is urgent.

On holiday

If you've got a family holiday on the horizon, or are planning an extended stay with family or friends, you may be wondering about whether to hold off on potty training until you're back home; or, if you've started already, perhaps you're worried how your toddler will manage while you're away.

Thinking about timing

You may be itching to start potty training, especially if your little one is showing signs of readiness (see p12), but if a holiday away from home is just round the corner, it's sensible to wait until you're back. You can tell your toddler that when you get back after the holiday he can try out some big boy pants, making this something to look forward to.

If you've started potty training, it's likely that at some point you will have to cope for a period of time away from home. The reality is that your toddler is likely to have more accidents in a new environment and potty training may regress. However, consistency is key, so although routines will be disrupted, as far as possible try to continue as you have been, and don't be too dispirited if accidents are more frequent. If you're holidaying somewhere warm, let your toddler run around with few, if any, clothes or pants on, so accidents are less of an issue.

Helpful preparation

If your toddler hasn't yet progressed to using a toilet, it's not a good idea to try this out first on holiday. Using a toilet is an adjustment for him, and it's best for him to do this is the comfort and familiarity of his own home. You can take his regular potty with you (or a travel potty, see opposite), or check out the facilities at your destination – perhaps they can provide a potty.

If your toddler has started to use the toilet, he will probably have to use various public toilets in transit and while away, which may feel strange and uncomfortable. Prepare him by getting him used to using different toilets in the weeks before you leave. Encourage him to try out toilets at friends' houses, in cafés, and in shops, so that by the time you go away, using unfamiliar toilets will seem normal. If he's unsure, use the toilet first, telling him you think it's fun to try a new loo! Alternatively, you could pack a portable toilet seat, which sits on top of a regular toilet seat. Or some travel potties double up as toilet seats. Get him used to using this before the holiday, so it will be familiar to him when you're away.

Getting there

Travelling to your destination with your potty-training toddler can be one of the most stressful parts of your holiday. It's best to be well prepared.

Make sure you have spare clothes, pants, and even shoes for your toddler, as accidents are quite likely on the way. Plastic shoes are ideal for travelling in.

Build in regular toilet breaks on your journey, even if your toddler doesn't seem to need to go. Young children often don't realize until the last minute that they need the loo, and may find that they do actually feel the need for a wee once you stop. If you're flying, take him to the loo before you board. A collapsible travel potty may be handy in your hand luggage, and will also be useful when you're out and about at your destination.

While you should give your child drinks, especially if requested, as you don't want her to become dehydrated, avoid giving him too much fluid en route, as this will inevitably mean more toilet stops. And steer clear of fizzy drinks, as these stimulate the bladder, so will make him need to wee even more frequently.

Some parents choose to use pull-up nappies for long journeys, and you may decide this is the easiest, most hassle-free path for you. This can work if you make it clear it's for the journey only and that he will switch back to pants when you arrive. However, it's good to avoid this as he could get used to wearing a nappy again, which will undo the good work he has been doing.

Limit the clear up en route by putting a waterproof mat under your child's seat in cars, trains, and on planes; or for an older child, use a special "travel" cushion to limit the impact of accidents.

If your toddler does have an accident, don't overreact. Of course, accidents add to the stress of a journey, but getting annoyed will simply make things worse. Appreciate that your toddler is out of his usual routine and isn't being lazy – holding on while travelling will be challenging for him. Remind him to let you know when he needs the loo, and reassure him that there will be plenty of toilet stops along the way.

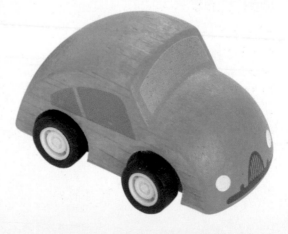

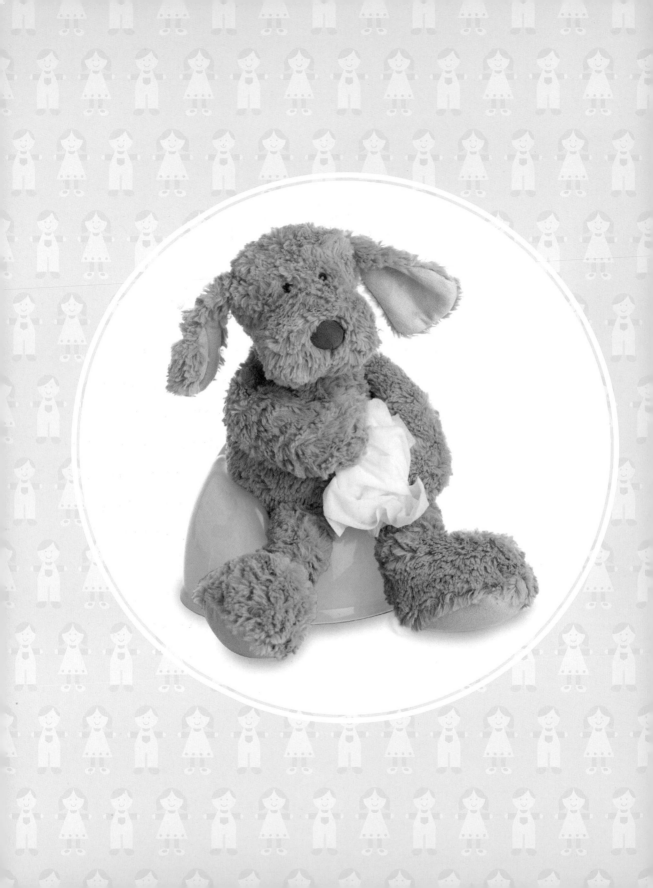

5

Problems along the way…

The path of potty training rarely runs smoothly. Whether it's the puddles and mishaps of the early weeks, slow progress over the months, or even coming to an abrupt stop just when everything seemed to be on track, there's a reason why potty training is often cited as one of the more stressful aspects of early years parenting! While you may be told by well-meaning friends not to worry, and that you are unlikely to see your child starting school in nappies, it's helpful to know how to deal with common setbacks, so that you and your little one can reach your goal in as calm a frame of mind as possible.

Dealing with accidents

Learning to use the potty is an acquired skill, just like learning to crawl, walk, and talk. Your toddler didn't simply stand up one day and walk without taking any tumbles. Similarly, potty training takes time and loads of practice, which means that a few accidents are usually inevitable as she learns this skill.

Understanding why accidents happen

Toddlers usually need to urinate around four to eight times a day, and can pass a stool around one to two times a day (although some have more or fewer bowel movements). This means there are plenty of opportunities for your little one to miss getting to the potty in time, and accidents are likely for at least the first six months while your toddler adjusts to her new potty routine. Still, it can be hard for grown-ups to put themselves in their toddler's shoes and understand why he or she can't get to the potty on time, which seems like a relatively simple task to them.

Bear in mind that to make it to the potty each time she needs a wee or a poo, your toddler first needs to recognize and pay attention to the sensation that her bladder or bowel needs emptying. Then she needs to focus solely on this so that she can plan to get to the potty in time to get undressed and sit on it. Expecting your child to process this information

every time she needs her potty and to carry it through successfully each time from the outset is unrealistic; your toddler is only just getting used to having control over her bladder and bowel, and in the early days of potty training she won't be able to hang on for very long.

Potty training can be challenging, but being mentally prepared helps you to take things in your stride.

Furthermore, young children can find it quite challenging to prioritize a certain piece of information, so if your toddler is engrossed in another activity, she may find it difficult to pay sufficient attention to the sensation of needing to wee or to poo, and may simply not notice that she needs to get to her potty.

What you can do

While accidents are to be expected, sometimes there are reasons behind them that can be addressed:

• When your toddler is overtired, she may be less likely to pay attention to signals that she needs the loo, and might not be able to hold on long enough to get to her potty. Make sure she isn't missing out on essential naptimes.

• If your toddler is very excited, or very absorbed in what she is doing, she may forget to use her potty, so keep an extra close eye on her during these times.

• If you are away from home, your toddler may find it hard to cope with her toilet needs in a different environment. Or a change to her routine such as moving home, a new baby in the house, or starting at a new playgroup, may unsettle her and throw her off her potty routine. Be extra vigilant during times of change.

Mopping up

You may be understandably anxious about your soft furnishings once your toddler starts potty training! The trick is to deal with accidents quickly to avoid stubborn stains developing. Get your toddler clean and dry first, then sponge carpets or chairs with cold water, working from the centre out. Carpet and furniture shampoos can also be effective.

• Toddlers have bad timing! Often, they leave going to the potty to the very last minute, and then fail to make it on time. Keeping an eye on her and reminding her regularly to use the potty can help.

• Your strong-minded toddler may resist using the potty if she feels pressure from you to use it (see pp66–7). Being relaxed and patient can take the tension out of potty training.

• Be alert to signs your toddler needs the loo: is she squirming, clutching herself, or jumping up and down in the classic "toilet dance"? If so, ask her if she needs her potty, or take her to the toilet yourself.

Started too soon?

If your toddler seems to be having an accident almost every time she needs the loo, it's possible she's not quite ready for potty training. If progress is virtually non-existent from the start, it might be worth stopping potty training for two or three weeks, or longer, then having another go later on.

Your response to accidents

While potty-training accidents are fairly unavoidable, how you react to these mishaps can be key to how smoothly potty training goes. Staying calm when your child has an accident and gently praising her achievements will help her confidence to grow, while reacting with annoyance, or even anger, could knock her self-esteem and result in setbacks.

Make a concerted effort to be patient. Inevitably, there will be occasions when managing to keep your cool will be more challenging, for example when you're all set to leave on a family outing and your toddler wets her best dress. However, losing your temper will simply exacerbate the situation: you will feel doubly stressed and your toddler may start to feel anxious and fearful about potty training generally, which could lead her to resist, and even rebel, against the process.

Getting cross might also make your little one feel shame and a sense of failure, neither of which are helpful emotions for potty training. And don't ever punish your child for a toilet accident, or tell her that she's old enough to know better. It's unlikely she has acted on purpose, so this reaction from you will be confusing and upsetting for her. Remind yourself that having accidents is

Respond to accidents gently and with plenty of understanding.

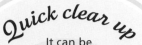

Quick clear up

It can be tempting to throw soiled pants away rather than attempt to clean them. A good tip, though, is to give them a quick "prewash" by holding them inside the toilet bowl while you flush, which will hopefully wash away most of the stool, then pop the soiled pants in the washing machine.

Try to take accidents in your stride and simply accept these are part of your life for the next few months.

a normal part of the learning process for her, and will help her to move forwards as she learns to read and react to signals more quickly in future.

Don't let your child spend long in wet or soiled clothes. While it's useful for her to recognize that she's wet or soiled – which she may not do if you whisk off her clothes within seconds of an accident – do change her promptly and without a fuss.

And remember to be loving. Leaving nappies behind is a big step for your toddler, so giving her a reassuring cuddle and telling her not to worry when she has an accident, and that she can try to get to the potty next time, will help her feel loved, supported, and, importantly, motivated to succeed in future.

Bowel movements

Using the potty to poo can take some getting used to as it's a very different sensation to doing a poo in a nappy. Some children refuse to use the potty at first for bowel movements, insisting on using a nappy still. It's best to accept this, then gradually work towards your child doing a poo in her potty. First, suggest she sits on it with her nappy on while she does a poo. You could also show her how you flush poo from her nappy down the toilet, so she understands how this happens. Eventually she will use the potty for all her toilet needs.

Bowel accidents can occur if she is constipated (see pp92–3) or has loose stools. When constipated, stools harden and are uncomfortable, or painful, to pass. Your child may hold back on using the potty, then when she is unable to hold on any longer, will lose control and has an accident. Check her diet and that there's no anxiety around potty training.

If she is feeling unwell, has drunk too much juice or eaten lots of fruit, her stools may be loose and she will be less aware she needs the potty.

Deal with bowel accidents calmly, as you would when she wets herself. Reassure her that it's nothing to worry about, and let her see you flush the poo away in the toilet where it belongs.

Slow progress

After an enthusiastic start to potty training, your patience may start to wane if your toddler's progress seems to be grindingly slow. Your frustration may double if friends' children seem to breeze through the whole potty-training programme with few apparent hiccups. Try to contain your feelings, avoid comparisons, and focus instead on thinking about the best way forward.

A loss of motivation

Potty training can be hard work at times for your toddler. Not only is she learning a complex new skill, she also has to practise it constantly and try to do it perfectly each time she needs to empty her bladder or bowel. While taking a tumble when learning to walk was upsetting for her, she could usually pick herself back up quickly and carry on. Learning to use the toilet involves following through all the steps required, as well as remembering to

Motivating yourself
Potty training
may be starting to feel
like a slow and painful marathon, but
try not to let this dampen your motivation
to support your child. Just as you didn't
give up encouraging her to master the art
of walking, despite numerous stumbles,
so you should continue supporting
her to master potty training –
she'll get there eventually.

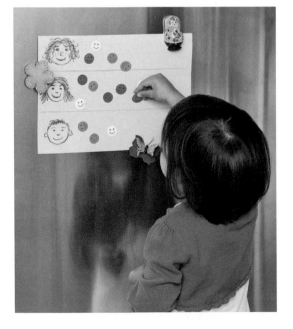

wipe herself, get dressed again, and wash her hands. And while she is getting to grips with all of these steps, potty training can seem like an uphill struggle. For some children, keeping this going can be too much, and after the initial desire to please you wears off, her consistency may falter.

If you feel this could be the case, perhaps your child needs a new motivation to make the effort seem worthwhile. Has your praise for her efforts diminished so that she no longer feels there's any reward for her hard work? While praising constantly can prove wearing for you, and may also lose effectiveness, remind yourself that she is on a learning curve, so it's worth telling her regularly how well she is doing, and how soon it will all feel much much easier. Or you might decide she needs something more solid than praise. If you haven't yet tried a reward system (see p45), this could be the perfect time to put one in place. Whether stars, a sweet treat, or a special story, you may find that this added incentive is exactly what is needed to reignite your little one's interest.

Remind yourself that your toddler has only just started to gain control over her bladder and bowel muscles.

Reality check

You may be thinking that after weeks or months of potty training, surely your toddler should have got the hang of things by now. However, potty training is usually a slow process with ups and downs and only a few achieving "overnight" success. If you're beginning to feel exasperated by the lack of progress, perhaps you need to check that your expectations aren't too high. Are you being realistic? For most, becoming completely potty or toilet trained can take anything from three to 12 months, with those starting earlier usually taking the longest to train fully. You can't force your child to meet this milestone before she is really ready: only she can control her bladder and bowel. In the meantime, letting your frustration show is likely simply to dent her confidence.

Staying positive

If your toddler's accidents are wearing you down and you feel you're losing perspective, try to regain focus:

• **remind yourself** that accidents are normal. You don't expect your toddler to never spill a drink or take a tumble, so the same applies to using the potty – sometimes she won't make it.

• **don't lose confidence** in your parenting ability, which can happen all too easily! The fact that potty training is taking months doesn't mean you are getting it wrong: it's simply how potty training works.

• **avoid making comparisons** with other children: each child is different, and taking her time to potty train isn't a reflection on your child's general abilities. If others make unhelpful comments, try to ignore them, or simply explain that your child is learning to use the potty at her own pace, and you're happy she will get there when she's good and ready.

Your wilful toddler

Your little one's world is opening up as she gains mobility, agility, and her language skills grow. But as she strives for more independence, you may find at times you need to avoid getting locked into a battle of wills when she wants to control events. Some toddlers are particularly wilful, which can make potty training especially tricky.

Keeping your cool

It can be hard to conceal your annoyance if your little one continues to have frequent accidents when you feel she really should know better. If she is extremely uncooperative,

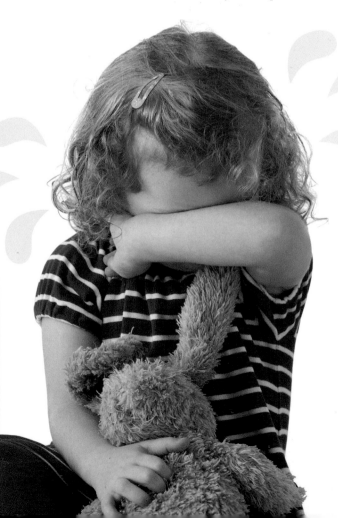

it might be better to wait a while to potty train until she is more ready and willing to have a go. If, though, you think she is ready and you would like to get started, try to find ways to work with her. Think about what could be going on in your toddler's mind. As she strives for independence, potty training (along with eating, another classic source of power struggles) is one of the few areas where she has some control – you can't make her empty her bladder or bowel in the right place at the right time. If you respond with annoyance or anger to accidents, a wilful toddler may sense that she has some control over your emotions, and toilet accidents could become a way of

> *Keeping a check on your responses can help to avert potty-training power struggles.*

gaining your attention, albeit not in a constructive manner. Moreover, a stubborn child is more likely to resist your requests when faced with your anger. If she is clearly testing boundaries, simply reset these calmly as you would with any other misdemeanour.

However, pretending to your child that everything is fine when it's not isn't necessarily the answer either. Your child may sense your annoyance and feel additional pressure to perform. While you don't want to admonish or punish her, it can be helpful to let her know calmly how you're feeling. Tell her that you are feeling a bit cross and tired today because you are having to do a lot of wiping up. This way she can understand why you aren't very happy, and that it isn't good to have wet or soiled pants, but she won't feel chastised. By not losing your temper you can avert power battles. For an older toddler, or one who is fairly well into potty training, you could also give her a cloth and request matter of factly that she helps you to clear up. This could be a good incentive to make it to the potty next time!

A consistent approach

A strong-willed child often likes to test limits, so it's especially important to be consistent when trying to gain her cooperation. Make sure that you, and anyone else who cares for her, such as a childminder or grandparents, follow the same approach to potty training. Let other carers know your programme: whether you prompt your little one to sit on the potty, or let her lead the way, and ensure that you have the same response to accidents.

This way, your child will know that everyone is working to the same plan, which will help her feel a sense of security and make her less likely to resist. With time, she will come to accept using the potty as a normal part of her routine and the appeal of resisting will fade.

Controlled choices

One easy way to avoid a battle of wills with your toddler is to give her more control over her situation. Some independence is what she is striving for, so letting her feel that she has made a decision can help to defuse her frustration and make her happier to do certain things. Perhaps you could ask her if she wants to use her potty upstairs or downstairs. Or whether she would like to use the potty before you read her a story or while you're reading to her. Of course, there may still be accidents, but she will feel that this potty-training business is something that she has a say in, too.

If your toddler really resists using the potty, perhaps you need to consider a more child-led approach (see pp14–5), letting her start potty training when she wishes to rather than when you would like her to start.

Common concerns

Whatever your potty-training journey, it's more than likely you will encounter a few hiccups along the way. Often, problems or scenarios you imagine you are facing alone are all too common, and it can be helpful to know that plenty of other parents encounter similar situations. Invariably, setbacks can be overcome with time, patience, perseverance, and some understanding.

My child uses the toilet at preschool, but wants a nappy on at home

You may feel frustrated and a bit confused if your child manages to use the toilets at preschool, but insists on reverting back to wearing a nappy at home.

This may seem nonsensical to you, but there's no point trying to reason with her. Try to think about the progress she is making rather than focusing on what she isn't managing. She is coping with a new school environment, including using the toilets there. She is probably tired once she gets home, and perhaps feels she can relax better in nappies. As she gets used to school, she should gradually be able to cope both at school and home.

My child soils her pants repeatedly

It's not uncommon for a child to use the potty consistently for a wee, but resist using it for a poo (see p63), instead soiling her pants.

If this is happening, check first that your child is not constipated (see pp92–3). She may be holding on if bowel movements are painful, then having accidents when she loses control. If you think this might be the case, take dietary and lifestyle steps.

Some children are fearful of pooing in the potty or toilet at first (see p49). It's best to let them do it their own way, using a nappy if they wish, until their confidence grows.

My child struggles to communicate her needs

If a child is a slow developer in one or more areas, this may have an impact on how she copes with potty training.

Some parents find that children who take longer to develop language skills are late potty trainers, although this isn't always so. As communication is an important part of potty training, a child who struggles to express her needs may find it harder to cope, but don't assume this will be the case.

If there's an area she struggles with, perhaps coordination or speech, be ready to offer extra support with potty training.

Illness has set back my child's potty training

Potty-training setbacks can occur for a variety of reasons. If your child has been, or is, unwell, this is likely to cause her to regress.

Parents sometimes fail to make the connection between a recent or developing illness and continued accidents. Bear in mind that your child's routine is thrown off track when she's unwell, and it may take her a week or so to regain her equilibrium.

It's best, if possible, to avoid putting your child back in nappies or pull-ups, although if she has severe diarrhoea and/or sickness, this may be helpful for a couple of days.

How you are coping

How you handle potty training can impact on your child's progress. If life is busy and you are finding the frequent messes and clear ups stressful, your little one is likely to pick up on your stress and become anxious, and maybe even resistant to potty training. If you're struggling to cope, try to take a step back and think about ways to make the process easier.

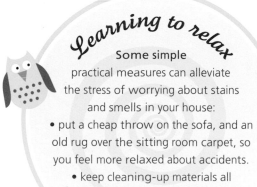

Learning to relax
Some simple practical measures can alleviate the stress of worrying about stains and smells in your house:
• put a cheap throw on the sofa, and an old rug over the sitting room carpet, so you feel more relaxed about accidents.
• keep cleaning-up materials all together so everything is to hand in one place when needed.

Not just one

While it's best not to start potty training just before a new baby is due, there are of course occasions when it's hard to get the timing right. Perhaps you potty trained your child successfully at the start of your pregnancy, only to find she regresses after the birth – a fairly common scenario when a new sibling arrives.

A new baby is a big change to your toddler's family setup, and at first represents a rival for your attention, as well as creating upheaval in your toddler's routine. Having realistic expectations about how she might respond will help you to feel mentally

prepared and avoid a build up of stress. If she does regress with potty training, reassure yourself that this is unlikely to last for long and is an understandable reaction.

Think about practical steps you can take to make life easier for you and your toddler. For example, you could place her potty next to your usual breastfeeding spot to keep an eye on her when you're feeding, praising her when she makes it to her potty. Carrying your baby in a sling around the house at times will allow you to spend time paying attention to your toddler, happy that your baby is secure. And don't feel guilty about putting your baby down in the safety of her cot occasionally so you can help your toddler with wiping or dressing, or to change her after an accident. Of course, if your partner, mum, or a friend is around, they can help to ease the load.

Be prepared for your toddler to regress a little with the arrival of a baby.

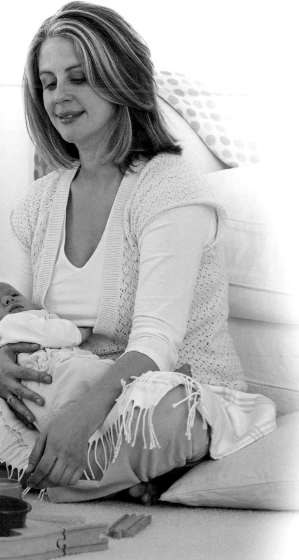

Working parents

If you work part- or full-time, you may wonder how on earth you will cope with potty training, or, if you've started potty training already, may be finding it a struggle when you return home tired, only to deal with accidents and a pile of washing.

The key to successful potty training while working is clear communication with your child's carer. If your child is yet to start potty training, you and her carer can check together the signs that she is ready and agree when it would be best to start. Your child's carer may prefer you to start off potty training when you have a run of free days, perhaps over a long weekend, then she can continue to work with you from that point. Make sure that your child's carer is aware of your approach so you both use the same cues, praise in the same manner, and deal with accidents in a similar way. If your child is at a day nursery, check their standard practice – perhaps they have hourly potty breaks – so that you can replicate this routine at home.

If you are using a reward system with your child, tell her carer about this, explaining how it works, and ask her to use it too. Agree together to let each other know about your child's progress, so that you can praise your child for how well she is doing with her carer when you're not there. This consistent approach will help your child to feel secure, supported, and confident about using the potty, and, handled well, she can bask in the praise of the very important people in her life: her parents and her carer.

Coming to a halt

Potty training can be unpredictable, and sometimes, just when you think your little one has finally got the hang of it, things take a turn for the worse and you wonder if you're back at square one! What should you do if potty training progress seems to have come to an abrupt halt?

Why toddlers regress

Your little one has been doing extremely well with her potty training, perhaps having just a couple of accidents a week, and you're congratulating yourselves that potty training has been a resounding success. Then she starts to have daily accidents, and you wonder what happened to all that progress.

Rest assured that potty-training regression is not at all uncommon. As with much of your child's behaviour, understanding how her world works can help you to work out why she is behaving in a certain way and think about what you can do to support her and get her back on track.

Even a small change in your child's routine can sometimes be enough to throw her off track.

When we learn a new skill as an adult, we are used to retaining the new information and being able to draw on it when needed. For children, however, it's not uncommon to move one step forwards and two steps back. Your child is learning in every area of her life, which although thrilling, can also be challenging at times, and sometimes a change to routine or an outside stress can be enough to throw her and cause her to regress in one area.

If your child's progress in potty training seems to have

halted, think about what is going on in her life. Often there's an obvious cause for potty-training regression; for example, you have moved house, your child has a new carer, or is starting a new nursery class. Sometimes, it takes just a relatively minor change in circumstance to cause your child to regress, such as moving to a big bed, or you or your partner getting a new job.

What you can do

Once you think you've identified the cause, talk to your child about what is happening and encourage her to tell you how she feels. Some children find it hard to articulate emotions, in which case talk to her gently about the changes that are happening in her life, and let her know that it's perfectly understandable that she has had more accidents recently. Reassure your little one that things will settle down soon enough and that you are confident she will get back on track with her potty training.

Back to nappies?

It's best to avoid returning to nappies, unless as a last resort, as this can be confusing and undermining for your child. Continue to support her with her potty training, making sure you are praising her for her efforts and giving her plenty of love and hugs. Sometimes, reinstating a previous reward system can be a great motivator (see p45). Think, too, about whether there is anything you can do to help ease her anxiety, such as talk to her nursery teacher about how she is feeling, or make sure she is surrounded by

Cause for concern

If you can't identify any particular stress factor in your child's life and feel puzzled as to the reason for her regression, it might be worth checking that there isn't a physical cause behind it. Sometimes, a condition such as an urinary tract infection or constipation (see pp92–3) can make going to the toilet an uncomfortable experience for your child. Ask your health visitor or doctor for advice if you're concerned.

familiar things in her new home. Let her know that you are sure she will get over this setback and that you will help her to carry on with her potty training, and, importantly, reassure her that you aren't feeling cross with her about accidents.

Occasionally, if a child is particularly stressed, you may decide it's best for her to have a break from the potty altogether. If, though, you can avoid doing this and persevere with potty training, accepting that things are moving a little more slowly than you would like, this may be the best course of action. Having to start almost from scratch again some time in the near future could be stressful and difficult for everyone involved. Remember, whichever course you choose, try to focus on the fact that whether earlier or that little bit later, eventually your child will succeed in mastering the potty.

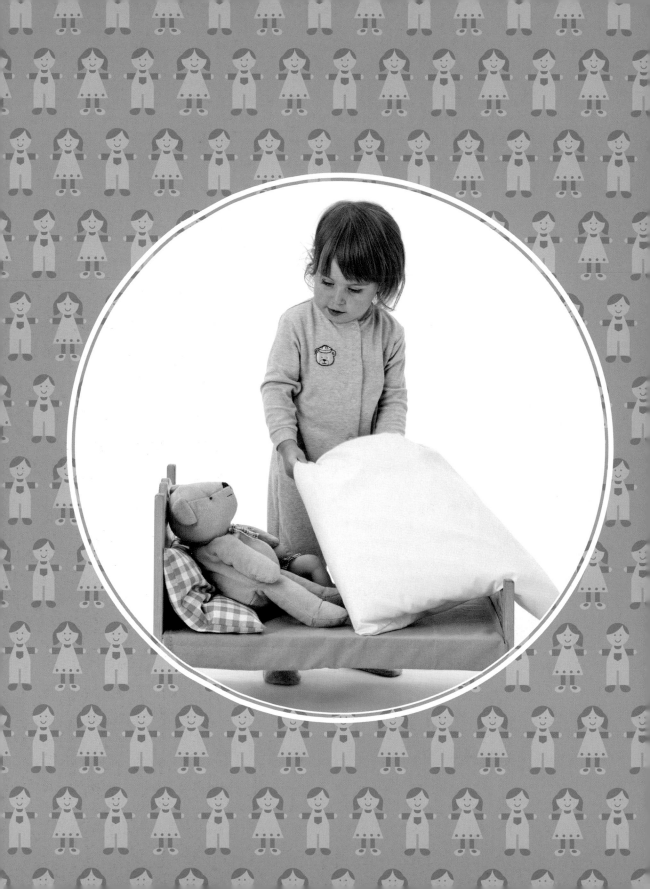

6
Dry nights

Your clever toddler is clean and dry during the day now, and you're delighted to have dispensed with nappy changes. Nighttime dryness usually comes later, as your toddler's bladder muscles need to be sufficiently developed for him to stay dry for a whole 10 to 12 hours. While you may be keen to ditch nappies for good as soon as possible, trying to rush this step could be counterproductive. As with daytime dryness, waiting until you spot signs that your little one is physically ready has the advantage that when he does go nappy free, he's more likely to master the challenge. It's probably realistic not to expect overnight success. For some children, the process is gradual and happens in fits and starts – although others are dry in just a few nights and never look back.

The next step

Your toddler has mastered staying dry during the day – well, perhaps there's the occasional accident – and you may wonder if the next logical step is to say goodbye to nappies at night. In reality, it may be a while yet before his bladder is strong enough to hold on all night, but you can start to watch for signs that he might be ready.

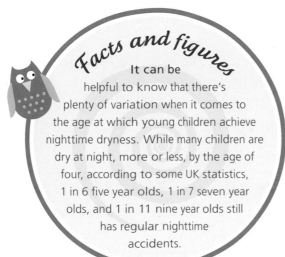

Facts and figures

It can be helpful to know that there's plenty of variation when it comes to the age at which young children achieve nighttime dryness. While many children are dry at night, more or less, by the age of four, according to some UK statistics, 1 in 6 five year olds, 1 in 7 seven year olds, and 1 in 11 nine year olds still has regular nighttime accidents.

Nights without nappies

It doesn't automatically follow that once your child can stay dry during the day, he should be able to manage to hold on throughout the night. If your toddler regularly wakes with a wet nappy, and still needs to wee every couple of hours during the day, it's unlikely that he is ready to cope without nappies at night. Most children do manage to stay dry at night by the age of four; and for those who took to daytime potty training with few problems and perhaps relatively early, say before 24 months, nighttime dryness might follow on shortly after. However, nighttime accidents

are still likely, and indeed considered perfectly normal, up to the age of five.

Staying dry at night requires far more control than staying dry during waking hours. To get through the night without using a nappy, your little one needs to sense while asleep that his bladder is quite full, and then either manage to hold on instinctively while he sleeps, or respond by getting up in the night to go to the toilet or use his potty. For some children, holding on during daytime naps isn't always easy, so managing to do this for 10 to 12 hours during the night is a big challenge. In the meantime, while his bladder is continuing to mature, your toddler will carry on weeing throughout the night quite unaware that he is doing so.

When is your child ready?

Over time, your child's bladder capacity will increase and he'll reach the point where he can hold on throughout the night, or where the urge to go is strong enough that it succeeds in waking him up in time for him to go to the loo. Some children, usually older ones, may decide themselves that they no longer want to wear nappies at bedtime – often motivated by older siblings or other children – and are keen to try to get through the night without them.

Even if your child doesn't show a particular interest in dropping nighttime nappies, you can watch out for signs that he is ready to make this step (see below). If you can see that he is dry for long periods of time in the day, you may need to take the initiative and suggest he could try to go without nappies at night, and get up to go to the toilet if he needs to do a wee.

When your child does start to go without nappies at bedtime, it's quite normal for it to take a while before he can manage to stay dry reliably each night, so bear this in mind and don't expect quick success, or worry that he is lagging behind friends. As with staying dry during the day, dry nights are something your child will achieve in his own time, and indeed can only achieve when his bladder is sufficiently mature.

The following are an indication that your toddler might be ready to manage staying dry during the night:

• On several occasions he has had a dry nappy first thing in the morning, or wakes up with a nappy that's wet but warm, suggesting he has held on almost all night and only just had a wee.

• He wakes during the night when he needs the loo, perhaps calling out to you, and maybe letting you know that he needs to do a wee.

• He manages to stay dry for longer periods of time during the day, stretching to three, or sometimes four, hours.

Getting started

Your little one is showing the signs that he is ready to go without nappies at night (see p77), so it's time to get started. As with daytime dryness, ensuring that your toddler is emotionally prepared, as well as being physically ready, will help everything to run as smoothly as possible.

Talking it through

Before you first introduced the potty, you did plenty of preparatory work with your toddler, talking to him about what it was for, telling him why this skill was important, and getting him ready and motivated for this step. Of course, he is now fully aware of what going to the toilet is all about, but this doesn't mean he can move seamlessly to nights without nappies, so it's important to talk him through this next step, too.

When you think he is ready to go without a nappy at night, chat to him about this. Tell him you're proud of how well he's managed potty training so far, and that you think he may be ready to manage without any nappies. Explain that he may have a few accidents, but reassure him that this is normal and nothing to worry about. Ask him how he feels about taking this step, and make a plan for if he gets up in the night. The idea of waking in the dark and managing

A protective mattress cover will minimize the impact of accidents.

to go to the loo or use his potty alone can be a particularly daunting one, so it's important he is reassured you are all on board and that this is something you will manage together.

Let him know that it's perfectly fine to get up in the night to go to the loo, so he doesn't feel that he should stay in bed and hold on. Perhaps he would like to wake you so you can take him to the toilet, or would prefer to have a potty by his bed, so that he doesn't need to worry about leaving his bedroom. He may wish to call you even if he doesn't need to leave his room, as most young children need reassurance when they wake alone in the dark. He may simply want to tell you that he has got up and done a wee, and for you to tuck him back in.

Ready to start

Once you are happy that you and your toddler have decided on a plan, you can get started. Put a waterproof cover on his bed, explaining what this is for if he asks. Encourage him to go to the toilet before bedtime, building this in to his routine. Make sure, too, that he can make his way easily to the bathroom in the dark: is the hallway clear, and does he need a nightlight in his room so he doesn't stumble?

Sometimes he may wake in the night for no apparent reason. If this happens, suggest he visits the toilet or potty before he goes back to sleep – it may be a while before he makes the connection between waking and needing a wee.

Getting through the night

While getting through the night without an accident isn't likely to happen straight off, be sure to give him praise and encouragement

Being prepared

Have all you need in place before your toddler attempts to get through the night nappy free:

• **A washable waterproof** mattress cover can be invaluable. Many come with a soft cotton top layer and a breathable waterproof layer so that your toddler doesn't become sticky and uncomfortable and the cover doesn't rustle when he moves.

• **A nightlight** can be comforting and practical in your child's room, helping to guide him in the dark.

• **A potty next to the bed** can be helpful and reassuring when your toddler starts nights without nappies.

along the way: when he goes to the toilet before bedtime, if he wakes you to go to the loo, and of course whenever he does manage to get through the night dry. When he wakes in the morning, remind him to visit the loo first thing, whether or not he had a wee in the night. As with daytime dryness, your encouragement will be valued and can motivate him to keep trying. However, avoid putting pressure on him. While your praise is important, he can't control when he gets through the night dry, so the aim is for him to feel supported along the way, as well as rewarded for success.

Dealing with nighttime accidents

Nighttime bedwetting can continue for weeks, months, and sometimes longer. And as with daytime dryness, it seems that boys are more likely to have accidents than girls. Accepting that bedwetting is an expected part of the process and learning to minimize the impact of nighttime accidents will reduce anxiety and stress all round.

How to react

Getting used to nights without nappies is a big step for your little one. Not only is he learning to react to signals in the night that he needs a wee, he also has to deal with waking in the dark and getting to the potty or toilet, which may feel scary and bewildering. In the early days, you can expect accidents up to two or three times a week. But as his bladder gets stronger, he'll be able to hold on for 10–12 hours: for most children, accidents get less frequent over time, and by five years of age, the majority have accidents rarely, if ever.

Try to respond calmly to bedwetting. Feeling wet in the night and lying on a soaked sheet is unpleasant and distressing, and if your little one also senses your annoyance, he is likely to feel negative and despondent, which could lead to more bedwetting as his confidence dips. Responding to nighttime accidents as you did with daytime mishaps – as a natural and expected stage – will help your little one to get past any upset and keep trying. Avoid, too, expressing feelings of concern about his bedwetting, as this could make him feel anxious, and even affect his ability to hold on during the night.

Taking nighttime accidents in your stride will help to avoid your child becoming despondent.

If your child seems disheartened when he wets his bed, reassure him that this is simply a phase. A simple explanation of how the bladder fills like a balloon and then releases wee when it gets too full, and that his brain needs to tell him when this is about to happen, can help him to understand what is happening at night and that bedwetting is not his fault. Never be tempted to punish or reprimand him for wetting his bed. This is not something he can control, and being punished could be deeply upsetting for him.

Practical support

There are some practical things you can do to support him and help him gain control over his bladder at night:

• Give him regular fluids during the day, giving more earlier in the day and slightly less closer to bedtime. Reducing his fluid intake isn't recommended, though. It's important that he is properly hydrated, and if you reduce the amount he drinks, his bladder will simply adjust and feel full with less fluid. Drinking plenty helps him learn to respond to a full bladder, which in time will help him recognize

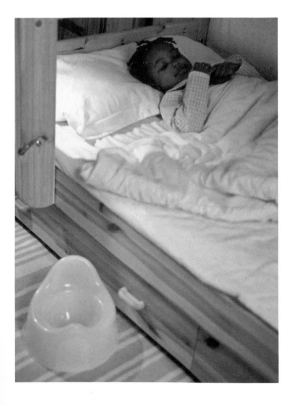

Lifting your child

Some parents help their child to avoid nighttime accidents by lifting them out of bed just before they head off to bed themselves, carrying their child to the toilet, then sitting them on the seat, or supporting boys if they stand, while they do a wee. There's no right or wrong about this, and some families find this is a good way to get through the night without mishaps. However, sitting your child on the toilet while he is half asleep doesn't teach him to recognize and respond himself to signals that his bladder is full, and may be encouraging him to wee in the night rather than learn to hold on. He is unlikely to remember going to the toilet with you in the night, and ultimately this could prolong the time it takes him to manage dry nights on his own.

signals from his bladder in the night, too.

• Avoid giving fizzy or caffeine-containing soft drinks, which stimulate the bladder.

• Ensure he visits the loo before bedtime.

• Offer encouragement, and praise him when he has a dry night.

Keep spare pyjamas and bed sheets to hand so you can change sheets and clothes in the middle of the night with minimal fuss. In the morning, a quick shower will keep him fresh and eradicate any lingering smell of urine that might be picked up on by other children.

When bedwetting continues

It's not uncommon for older children to continue to wet their beds, and around one in six five year olds still wets their bed regularly, which is known as nocturnal enuresis (see p93). As with any toilet accident, your constant support and reassurance will help your child overcome this phase.

Should you be concerned?

Just as your child had accidents when he first went without a nighttime nappy, continuing to wet his bed after the age of five is not something he can control or should be reprimanded for. Often, whether prolonged bedwetting is seen as a problem or not is down to your own perception. Perhaps you wet the bed yourself at school age and so feel relaxed that this is quite normal, and are confident that your child will soon grow out of it. Or you may be particularly concerned because your child's older cousins – or your friends' children – were dry at night by this age.

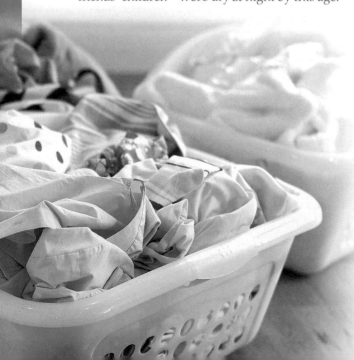

Prolonged bedwetting can be frustrating, but solutions can be found.

The point at which many parents become concerned is when bedwetting starts to interfere with their child's socializing. As your child gets older, he may become aware that friends no longer need nappies at night or wet their beds, which may cause him some anxiety and embarrassment when it comes to taking part in sleepovers, and he may even try to avoid these social occasions.

What causes prolonged bedwetting?

Often, continuing to wet the bed beyond the age of five is simply down to the fact that your child is taking a little longer to develop his full bladder response and is unable to hold the amount of urine produced during the night. For some children, the bladder's capacity is slightly smaller. There can also be a genetic link to prolonged bedwetting, and boys are twice as likely as girls to have nighttime accidents. Recent research suggests that bedwetting can occur when the body produces less of the hormone vasopressin, which reduces urine production in the night to enable a good night's sleep. Sometimes bedwetting can be caused by a problem such as constipation (see pp92–3), or, less commonly, a urinary tract infection (see p93), in which case your doctor can advise you on how to relieve the problem, or deal with an infection. It's important to understand that your child is not wetting the bed because he is being lazy or unhelpful, and that, with understanding and support, this phase will eventually pass.

A step back

Occasionally, a child who was previously dry at night regresses and starts to wet the bed again, a condition known as secondary nocturnal enuresis. This usually occurs in response to a stressful situation, for example, if you've recently moved house, or there's tension at home or at school. Think about what could be causing your child's stress, and then give him plenty of reassurance and loving support to ease his anxiety. If the cause isn't so obvious, it might be worth having a chat with his teacher to see if he or she has an idea of what it is that might be upsetting your child.

How to help

Continuing to support your child emotionally and letting him know that his nighttime accidents are not his fault will be immensely reassuring for your little one and will help to reduce any anxiety he feels, which in turn could actually start to relieve the problem. Continue, too, to offer plenty of practical support (see pp80–1), to both help prevent bedwetting incidents and to minimize the

When to get help

If bedwetting continues and you think that your older child's self-esteem is affected, you could talk to your health visitor or doctor about possible bladder training programmes or a bedwetting alarm, which can work well with older children. When your child starts to wee, an alarm is set off, prompting him to get up and go to the bathroom. Over time, his bladder becomes conditioned to responding when it's full.

Occasionally, doctors prescribe medication to suppress urine production at night, but this isn't usually a long-term solution. If you think your child has discomfort or difficulty when passing urine, wees excessively, or is very thirsty, talk to your doctor to rule out an underlying health problem. Online forums and helplines, provided by organizations such as ERIC (see p96), a charity that offers advice on childhood continence, give support and allow you to connect with other families in the same situation.

impact of them when they do occur. Special pyjama pants are available for older children who have a continued problem with bedwetting. These look like normal pants, but have a thin, very absorbent pad, so can help to save your child embarrassment at sleepovers or family get-togethers.

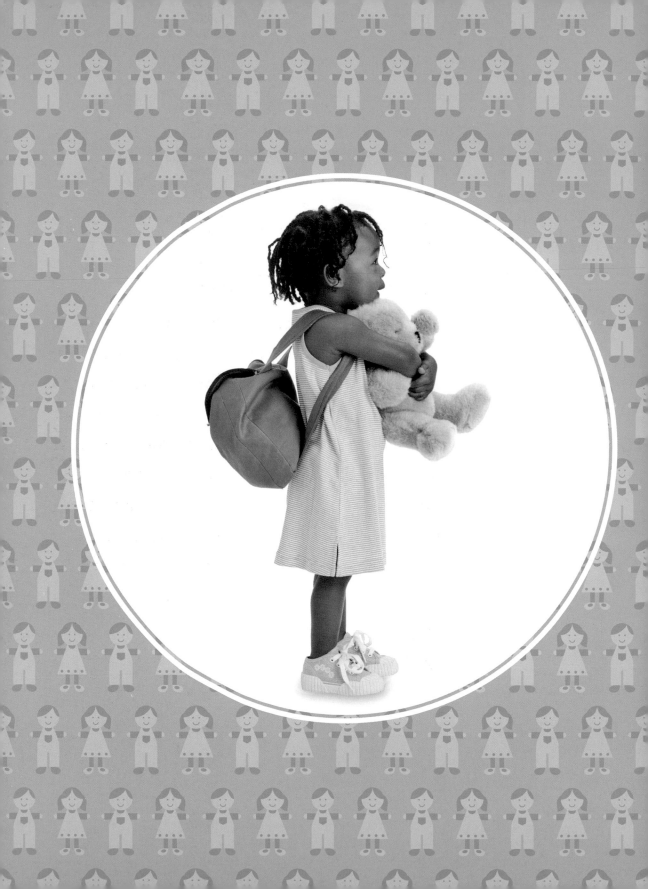

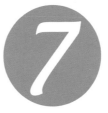

Special situations

Every family and every child is different, and there are times when you may need to adapt your approach to potty training to suit your particular circumstances. Whether your little one is due to start preschool and you're worried she's not quite ready; your child's time is divided over two households; or she has special needs that mean she requires a particular type of support, it's important to tune in to her individual requirements. It's useful, too, for parents and carers to be aware of medical conditions, such as constipation, that can affect how your child copes with potty training. Spotting the signs that something isn't quite right will mean you can quickly take steps to get your little one back on track.

Ready for nursery?

You're sure your child will get the hang of staying dry in her own time, but still you may feel pressure if she's due to start a nursery that asks for children to be toilet trained, for example a preschool for three to four year olds, in the near future. While potty-training "deadlines" are unhelpful, putting some thought into this now can help your child feel prepared.

Preparing for preschool

You may be getting worried about how your little one will cope with the toilet regime at preschool. However, conveying your concerns to your child is not a good idea. She doesn't have your understanding of timescales, and making her feel that she is on a schedule with a deadline for dryness is likely to make her feel stressed and even more prone to accidents. Starting preschool is a big step for her, so she needs to feel confident and supported, not worried about having accidents when she gets there.

Starting preschool is a big leap for your little one.

What's the policy?

Make sure you're clued up on the preschool's toilet-training policy. If you are still waiting for signs that your little one is ready to start potty training, talk to the nursery about how this will be managed. They may want your child to wear pull-up trainer pants at first. While it's best to avoid these, as the absorbency of pull-ups means your child may not always be aware when she has done a wee, you may have to compromise and accept that toilet training might take a little bit longer. Check out, too, the policy on bowel accidents. Will the school expect you or a carer to come in and help your child to change, or is this something they are prepared to handle? They may suggest that your child brings in a plastic bag with a change of clothes, with wet or soiled clothes taken home in the bag. Be open with the staff about what stage your child is at with toilet training, rather than hoping for the best. They will soon become aware of what your child is

Aim to visit the preschool a couple of times with your child before she starts. Check out the toilet facilities with her and talk to staff about how they manage toileting. If possible, ask if she can use the toilet while there (if she is ready to do this), so that it will be slightly familiar when she starts. The more informed both of you are, the better prepared she will be.

capable of, and if you're upfront with them from the outset, they will be able to provide the right level of aid and support to help your child settle in to her new environment.

Get into the routine

Finding out about the daily routine at preschool means that you can start to replicate this at home, which will help your child to feel more prepared when she starts there. For example, perhaps staff give half hourly reminders to children to use the toilet, or take them to the toilet at regular intervals, including set times such as before or after meals and before they play outside. Gently easing your child into a similar routine at home will help her to feel comfortable and familiar with how things work when she starts nursery, and, in the best-case scenario, may help her bladder adjust to this routine before she gets there.

Backwards and forwards

If your child has coped well so far with potty training and you're confident she will manage at preschool, you may be taken aback if she suddenly seems to regress a little once she starts. Remind yourself, though, that not only is she entering into a new environment, meeting new children and nursery teachers, but she's also having to adapt to a new routine, all of which equals a lot of change and is likely to wear her out. A temporary setback is no surprise. Be patient and talk to the teachers about how best to help and support your child. Perhaps she is worried about putting her hand up and asking to go to the loo, in which case, nursery staff could make sure that they check

Some children embrace change and respond well to their new toilet regime.

with her regularly to see if she needs to visit the toilet. If she seems tired, make sure she is getting sufficient rest at home so that she can cope better during the day.

You may find, though, that your child's toilet-training prowess actually comes on in leaps and bounds when she starts her preschool nursery. Being in an exciting and stimulating new environment and seeing her peers use the toilet may be the perfect motivation for her to finally get to grips with her toilet routine.

More than one household

Your child's routine may be split over two households for various reasons: perhaps she is with a childminder in the week, or at her grandparents' house, or you and your partner may be separated and she spends time with each of you. Whatever the situation, when it comes to potty training, you will need to think about how you will manage her routine between you.

On the same page

Potty training is a considerable learning curve for your child, so it's important that the people helping and encouraging her aren't giving her conflicting advice and instructions. When more than one person is involved in her care, a consistent approach to potty training can avoid problems. This doesn't mean that routines can't differ slightly, and in fact some variation could be helpful preparation for when your child has to cope with new situations, such as starting in a nursery class.

However, it is important that your basic approaches to potty training correspond, so, for example, accidents are dealt with sympathetically, pull-ups aren't used in one house when you are trying to get your child used to pants, and one of you isn't putting her on the toilet when she prefers the potty. Your child may be happier using the same type of

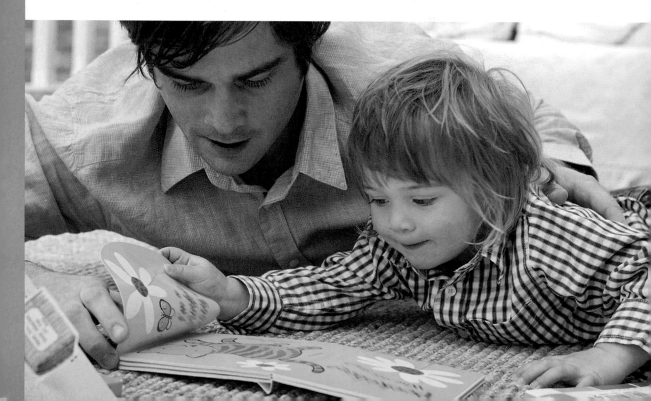

potty in different locations, as well as using the potty in a similar room in different houses, so perhaps always in the bathroom. Keep reward systems (see p45) consistent, too.

> *A consistent approach is key to keeping potty training on track.*

Carry on talking

Communication between carers is vital. Let each other know how your child is progressing and talk through problems or setbacks, so you can work together on solutions. Share, too, when your child has been doing well, so that if accidents happen while she is with her carer, she or he will realize this is a step backwards. Often, a perceived setback is simply a minor hiccup, but by discussing progress, problematic patterns can be spotted and addressed.

While you are in charge of how you potty train your child, being prepared to listen to and take on board others' advice can be worthwhile. Listening to an experienced childminder, especially if this is your first foray into potty training, can provide you with invaluable nuggets of advice.

Don't forget to check in with your child. Ask how she is coping with potty training in two households. Is she happy with the set-up in each house – perhaps there's something she prefers in one house? Is she confused about anything, or worried about upsetting a carer if she has an accident? Let her know that she can talk to you or her carer any time she has a concern.

When parents live apart

If you and your partner are separated, your child may be spending extended periods of time with you both, which may also involve spending nighttimes in more than one household. Even if relations between you and your partner are strained, it's important to try to put differences aside and form a united front to help your child through potty training. Decide on a strategy and agree to let each other know how she is getting on when she's with you. Try not to use potty training as a way to score points or criticize the other's approach as this will only cause tension and anxiety, which will make potty training harder for your child. She may even blame herself for your fall out. You may need to compromise at times too; for example, if your child spends weekends only with Dad, and he wants to take her out somewhere, this could be tricky with a toilet-training routine. Insisting that he stays in with her could cause resentment, so try to relax and accept that potty training may just take a little longer. Reassure your child that neither of you is cross if she has an accident, telling her, for example, that this won't spoil her weekend with Daddy. Seeing you agree and work together will help her relax and reassure her that she is well supported by you both.

Children with special needs

Mastering potty training is a big achievement for all children, and children with special needs especially benefit from this step towards independence. However, a child with physical or learning difficulties is likely to take much longer to potty train, and require plenty of patience and understanding.

Welcome support

As potty training a child with special needs can take longer, it's important to be prepared for this, and line up additional support if necessary. You and your partner can be mutually supportive, and you may need to enlist the help of your health visitor and specialists. Tell family and friends you are potty training so they can offer help and lift your spirits if needs be.

The best time to start

While some children with special needs may start potty training a bit later than usual, as with any child, deciding when to start potty training depends on the individual child and their signs of readiness. For example, if your child is staying dry for a couple of hours at a time, is aware when she has done a wee or a poo and can tell when she is wet, or seems motivated to start, then now might be the right time.

Depending on your child's needs, she may need more help in a particular area, for example, with getting undressed if coordination is a problem, so this needs to be considered. It can be worth tuning in to her

natural bowel and bladder patterns, too, so when she does start, you will have a sense of when she needs the potty.

As well as looking for physical signs, think about your child's personality to gauge how she might cope with potty training and how you can best support and motivate her.

Children with social learning difficulties

If your child has social learning problems, she may be resistant to change, so getting started with potty training could be a challenge. As with all children, think about how she responds best and which methods are most likely to encourage her. She may, for example, respond well to a potty routine and come to see this as an integral part of her day.

Often children with social learning difficulties are particularly sensitive to sensory stimulation, which can raise problems during potty training. For example, a child may dislike the feel of the potty, the smell of the toilet, or react badly to the sound of the toilet flushing. Being aware of potential pitfalls and listening to her concerns will mean you can make helpful changes, such as positioning the potty away from the toilet, or using a padded toilet seat instead of the potty if she finds this more comfortable. Starting off using the toilet might have benefits as your child won't have to make another adjustment later on from the potty to the toilet.

If she lacks the motivation to start, perhaps she simply isn't interested. You may need to wait a while longer, and watch instead for physical, rather than emotional, signs that your child is ready, such as the ability to stay dry for two or more hours, and showing recognition of when she is wet or soiled.

As with any child, support and understanding make a good foundation for potty-training success.

Children with physical difficulties

If your child lacks coordination, learning to use the potty or toilet can be especially hard, and a great deal of practical support and assistance may be required. You may need to get expert help on deciding when to start potty training your child, and how to teach her bladder and bowel control.

While you may be preoccupied with your child's physical struggles, it's important not to neglect preparing her emotionally for using a potty. Talk to her about this step, let her watch you use the bathroom, and offer support and praise whenever she succeeds, or simply tries.

Sight and hearing difficulties

A child with hearing or vision problems will have obvious challenges when it comes to mastering the potty. If your child has impaired hearing, and perhaps speech difficulties, too, communication – an important part of potty training – will be tricky. As well as employing your usual methods of communication, such as signing and gestures, place extra emphasis on visual cues, such as watching and observing others on the toilet and looking at colourful potty-training books together.

If your child is visually impaired, you will need to spend plenty of time explaining the process of using the potty to her, and taking practical measures such as ensuring that the potty is kept in the same place and that there are no obstacles to negotiate her way around on the way to the potty or bathroom.

Medical conditions

Occasionally, problems with potty training can be traced to a medical condition that makes it difficult for your little one to use the potty easily. If you have specific concerns about your toddler's bladder or bowel movements, talk to your doctor or health visitor for advice and reassurance.

Dealing with constipation

This isn't an uncommon problem in young children, and is caused by a number of interrelating factors. Constipation can develop if your child is anxious about using the potty for a poo, or feels pressure to get potty training right. Some children have particular fears about having a bowel movement in a potty, as they see their stool as an extension of their body and feel upset when it's flushed away. A child may insist on using a nappy still to do a poo, or otherwise may hold on when she feels the urge. Holding on means her stools gradually get harder and drier, which in turn makes passing a stool uncomfortable and even painful at times, and she may resist going to the toilet even more. Constipation tends to be more common in boys than girls at this age, possibly down to the fact that boys who stand to do a wee have to make a conscious decision to sit down to do a poo, and consequently may not do this as often as they should.

Constipation can usually be relieved through lifestyle measures. While young children shouldn't eat large amounts of fibre, as this fills up their small tummies without providing all the necessary nutrients, it's important for your child to have regular fibre to keep her bowels working well. This can come from fresh fruit and vegetables, dried fruit such as apricots and prunes, and wholemeal foods such as bread and pasta. It's important, too, for her to drink plenty of fluids, ideally water, but diluted fruit juice is fine, too.

Talk to your child's doctor if you're concerned about her bladder or bowel habits.

As well as diet, daily exercise will help to keep your child's bowel movements regular. Being constipated can cause sluggishness, but it's important to make sure that she has active periods each day.

If your child is in discomfort when passing a stool, applying some Vaseline around the base of the anus can ease this. If, despite a healthy diet, things don't ease, or your child has abdominal pain, vomiting, or hasn't had a bowel movement for days, get advice from

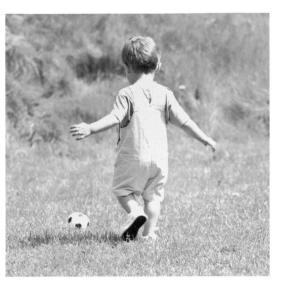

your doctor. Sometimes, a laxative may be prescribed, but you should never give these without consulting a doctor.

Urinary tract infections (UTIs)

These are more common in girls than boys as they can pass bacteria easily from the anus to the vagina while wiping. This is why it's important to teach girls to wipe from front to back, even after just a wee. UTIs aren't always easy to spot, but there are some telltale signs. They can affect bladder control, so if she's having more accidents than usual, perhaps feeling she needs the potty but not getting there in time, or she has a spate of accidents after a period of dryness, this may be the cause. Other symptoms include blood in the urine, pain while urinating, fever, and feeling generally unwell.

It's important to see a doctor if you suspect a urinary tract infection as your child will need a course of antibiotics to clear this up. Also, repeated infections can damage the kidneys, so symptoms shouldn't be ignored.

Elimination disorders

While accidents are an accepted part of potty training, repeated accidents over a period of time can be a concern. Enuresis is the term used for repeated wetting accidents after the age when this is considered normal, at around five years old. Enuresis can be nocturnal (see pp82–3), occurring at night, or "diurnal", occurring in the daytime, with nocturnal enuresis being the most common type. Encopresis is the term for repeated soiling.

If your child is having uncharacteristic accidents in the day, this can sometimes be caused by conditions such as an urinary tract infection (see left), or another underlying condition, which may need medical attention. Nighttime bedwetting is a common condition that usually improves as a child's bladder control matures, although long-term bedwetting can cause problems with self-esteem, so interventions may be useful (see p83).

Encopresis may be caused by chronic constipation (see opposite). When stools become very hard and impacted they may be too painful to pass. Some loose, more liquid, stool may then leak out past the bulky stool, which your child is unable to control.

Index

Acknowledgments

Publisher's acknowledgments

Dorling Kindersley would like to thank Claire Wedderburn-Maxwell for proofreading, and Michèle Clarke for the index.

All images © Dorling Kindersley. For more information see www.dkimages.com

Resources

www.eric.org.uk
Education and Resources for Improving Childhood Continence. Advice and information for parents on potty training and associated problems.

www.cafamily.org.uk
Support for families with children with disabilities.

www.familylives.org.uk
Parenting and family support with helpline and chat forum.

www.babycentre.co.uk
Online resource for new and expectant parents with chat forum.

www.mumsnet.com
Online forum for parents run by parents. Information and discussion threads on all aspects of parenting.

www.nct.org.uk
Childbirth and parenting charity with information on parenting.

www.tamba.org.uk
The Twins and Multiple Birth Association. Advice and support on raising twins.